How I Lost 100 Pounds

In 100 Days

Dexter Mason

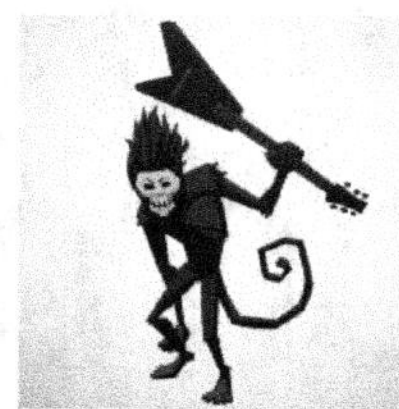

Table of Contents

Please Do Not Speedread Through This Book!

I know that we all can have the attention spans of a 2 year old at times. Especially in this fast paced, got to have it now world that we live in(snap – snap). But please, I am asking you to make my efforts in writing this book not be all for not, by you skimming through, or speedreading it. That will not serve you well, I promise. I really want you to read this book in a relaxed, calm frame of mind. You owe this to yourself. The information that I put together in this book is priceless. And I had to go through several hell's in my life in order to figure all of this stuff out. I am writing this book now, as I am in the best time of my life. The things that I say here, are really a watered down version of just some of the issues I was dealing with at this time. Sorry, but for my own health, I need it to be this way. Rather than dwelling on the past, and putting myself into a funk, as I write this book. I am choosing to not disclose every single detail about what my life was like at this particular time. This does not take anything away from the powerful message I am trying to get across inside of this book. The message I am trying to shout from the roof tops here, WILL add years to your life. And those years will be the most amazing years you can imagine. You will not find this message by skimming through the pages, looking for a miracle.

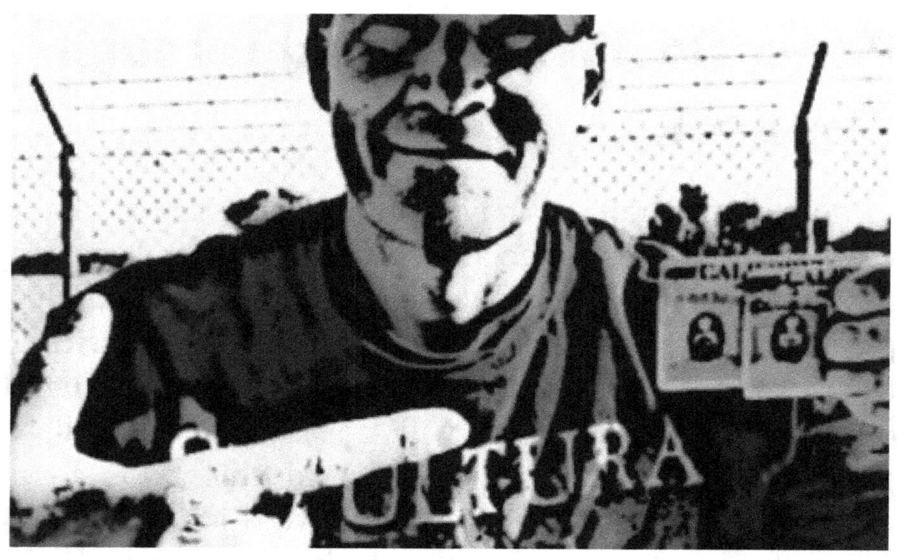

These are two of my old drivers licenses that I carry with me in my wallet. The one on the right, is from 2004, when I was 27. And the one on the left, is from 20006, when I was 29. I will keep these on my person for the rest of my life. Looking back now, I can see that the 20004 image was the tipping point, as to how much weight I could carry on my body, and not be a total fat mess. I was 275 lbs in that picture. And honestly about 10, Or 15 lbs over my limit at that time in my 20's, when I was able to hold a really large amount of muscle mass.

This is around the time when I let it all go, and eventually found myself weighing around 320 lbs. Which is where I was at in the 20006 photo. I have not looked at these ID photos in years. They just sit inside of my wallet, tucked away.

In fact, my original intent was not to ever even save them. But, out of laziness I suppose, I never threw them away. My plan was not to write this particular chapter in my life, until I was at least 50 years old. I have some reasons for this. But the other day, I just felt like looking at these old photos of myself, for no reason at all really? It was kind of surreal. I don't really know what made go into that little section of my wallet where I keep them, and look at them? Whatever it was, led me to being here now. Writing the intro to a book that I had not intended on writing for at least another decade. If I ever was going to write it at all. If you are reading this right now, then I obviously wrote it. So let me welcome you into my world for a bit, and share with you a part of me that I have never shared with anyone.

Brace yourself...

Ever since I was a small child. The two main goals that I had in life, were 1 - To one day become a 300+ pound, enormous hulk-like beast. Which I think many young boys have this goal, and can relate, even at a very young age.

And 2 - To commit suicide, in my very own special way. On my terms, and in some kind of memorable fashion that would draw attention to myself, while I am resting in peace.

As morbid as this sounds, it was true. And I felt this way ever since I could remember. I always had a fascination with my own death. Not others deaths, but my own. And it was not just some childhood phase I went through. As I carried this with me for the majority of the years that I have been alive. All the way up into my early 30's, when I had a **HUGE** transformation of my entire life.

Like I said, it was 1 of the two of my major goals in my life. I must be honest, and tell you that it will never fully get out of me. This demon that is inside of me. I am not "suicidal", nor was I ever "suicidal" in the typical sense of the word. I did not ever come off as that type of kid. But, I have always been really good at not letting others be affected (infected) by what goes on in between my own ears. I was, and still am proud of that attribute that I have.

I am the complete opposite of someone who likes to bring other people down along with them. I have always been a really respectful person, and have a natural common courtesy towards everyone. I was always very much in my own head. And was very content with staying to myself, and not needing any social status to make me feel good about myself.

I didn't really fit the "mold" of the typical introverted, shy, quiet type of kid that people have an image of in their heads. Even though I was all of those things. I still am those things. Being a quiet, lone wolf type of person, does not mean that you have something wrong with you. But, it doesn't mean that you don't either. We all have a lot of **something's** wrong with us. We are all humans. And we all must deal with issues.

How we deal with those issues, is what is most important.

When it came to my own issues. Well, I never really thought that I had any issues? **I had goals in life!** They were not issues to me until I got a little older. I eventually realized that my goals were going to lead to an early death, which is what I wanted right? Yea, it was. But I also wanted it to be on my terms.

I won't go into too much detail in this book, but I will possibly write another book on my past struggles with my fascination with my own death one day.

But since all of this intertwines with one another, I will speak about it on the surface. The day that I really can pinpoint, when I actually began to realize that my "goal" of suicide, was actually an "issue", that was harmful to me. Was when I came the closest that I ever have to achieving my life long goal. And this exact date was on January 1st, 2000.

Y2K

Remember that? The Y2K thing...

Well, I am going to make a very long, and painful story short. And tell you that I came very close to not seeing the 21st century happen. Very close. So close, that it actually woke me up from this delusional spell that I put my own self under. Well, sort of. It didn't turn my thoughts completely around, like they are now. But, it did make me realize that I had an issue on my hands. Did I immediately deal with that issues properly? No! Of course not. But in hindsight, I would not change anything about that time in my life. As if it had not happened the way that it did. I may still be under the spell of my own sick delusion, that I labeled as a life goal. Or worse. I may have achieved that goal, and not be here telling you about it now.

My Apology to You

In the beginning, I had mentioned that I have some reasons that I had not yet wrote this book. And that I had planned on writing it after I turned 50 years old, if I ever was going to write it at all.

Well, one of the reasons is this...

I am not the "fat kid".

And I never was the fat kid. I hope that you still will listen to my story, and use the information that I am giving you?

I imagine that most people reading this now, are, and were the "fat kid". This is one reason why I was planning on waiting until I was old enough to be respected for my thoughts, to write this out.

The "fat kid", might not want to listen to someone talk about weight loss, who also isn't the "fat kid". But I tell you that I did let myself get up to 320 lbs. And I was carrying way too much fat on my body for several years, before I decided to turn my life around.

I was always the athletic kid. I was very good at all sports, and EXTREMELY active. I was not skinny. But I was not fat. I had decent genetics for putting on muscle mass, especially on my lower body.

Like I mentioned earlier. I was able to hold 250, 260 lbs on my frame, while being athletic, and looking like a linebacker, in my early and mid twenties. I was squatting 500 lbs, and could still play basketball, tennis, football, run stadiums, and be an overall athletic young man. Those are just my genetics. But from about 260 lbs and up, I made a complete mess out of myself. 320 lbs was where I ended up, before I had even reach 30 years old.

This is why I rarely mention this, or have never written about it, in all of the books that I have written over the years. I never even tell people in the real world. Not even people who deal with their own weight issues. I just let them think that I am able to easily float around 190 – 200 lbs, with low body fat, and always have been. It is just easier for me to let this go on this way.

Another part of it is, that I am very mentally tough on my own self. And we will get into that later. But, I do not throw pity parties for myself. And I never have, even at my lowest of lows. It is not how I was raised, or even in my nature. My nature is to be too hard on myself to be honest. There is a balance there, and we all should strive to find it. But be honest about where that balance is.

Like I said, I am not the fat kid. I don't have fat kid issues. I have other issues. And they lead me to becoming 320 lbs.
I really want you to understand this. And understand that my 320 lbs, may not be you're 320 lbs. My obsession since I was a child, was to become 300 lbs. I made this a life goal of mine. I achieved it, and then some. So becoming huge was my thing. I was obsessed with it. I didn't ever get into the steroid thing, thank God. But, I did have the genetics to be able to put on thick amounts of muscle onto my legs, and butt mostly. But I was a comfortable 230 lbs, at a young age, and looked really good at that weight. If I were to weigh 230 lbs now, I would look fat, and not be in good health internally. I spent a decade trying to undo what I did. And have got myself to a comfortable position in life, where I can be under 200 lbs at all times.

As long as I continue to put my new obsession with vitality first. Because once we allow our body to become a specific weight once. We can always go back up to it again, if we lose sight what we should be focusing on.

My body doesn't really want to be 190 – 200 lbs. Even though I keep my weight there, without doing anything stupid to jeopardize my health. Please read that last sentence multiple times, and own it yourself. Never jeopardize your health, in order to be a specific weight on a scale.

My body actually wants to be about 210 lbs. I will be ok with that I guess if I had to be 210 lbs, although my quads, glutes, and hamstrings will be where that 10 – 20 lbs will go. But I feel amazing when I weigh under 200 lbs. And I even will sometimes get myself down under 190 lbs for a few days sometimes. Again, without doing anything to jeopardize my health. I do not "cut". I do not "bulk". I do not "bodybuild".

Do yourself a favor and try and forget all those internet terms. Think in terms of your own vitality. And turning the sands of time upside down. Grow younger. It is possible. I am living proof of it. And I show it with my blood work.

This is my dedication to everything that I love. Myself is now included in that category of everything that I love. And my self love must come first.

Yours must come first as well.

I made so many mistakes in the process of losing 100 lbs in 100 days. So many!

While I am speaking on that, let me tell you that I think I lied in the title. Ha! The title is just for effect, and it is a good eye catcher. 100 lbs, in 100 days. It just catches the attention of people looking to lose a lot of weight. This is why I chose to stick my own self on the cover, holding up my old photo ID's(cringe).

It takes a pair of brass ones to do that.

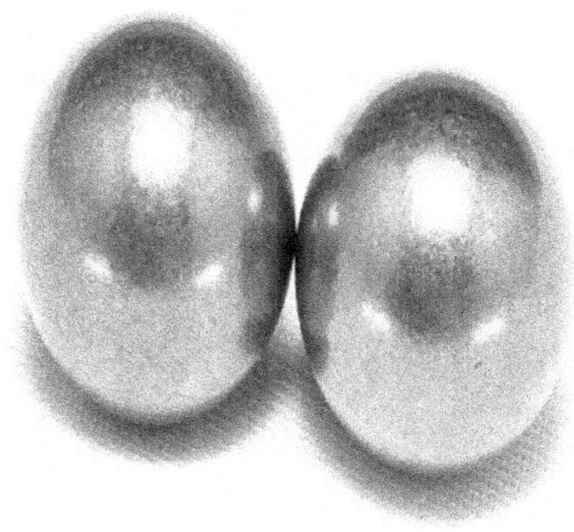

I think I actually lost 90 lbs, in 90 days, to be honest. And I eventually lost 130+ lbs in total. But the initial weight loss, I believe was around 90 lbs in 90 days. So, I apologize once again for that(not really…).

The reason that I am telling you this, and also the reason that I added a few pounds, and a few more days, which isn't a big deal. Is to kind of put less emphasis on the actual numbers themselves. Because they don't matter as much as overall health matters. That should always be the main focus. And any weight loss that comes with it, is a byproduct of the main focus.

The Bike Trail (Day of Reckoning)

This one day at the bike trail, was a very pivotal day in my life. It was a day that I finally had enough of the mess that I had made of myself. My younger brother of 11 years, had a huge role in this turning point for myself. He and I still laugh as we reminisce from time to time about this one very special summer day on the bike trail.

We laughed about it then as well. Even though it was at my expense. I deserved it, and I could do nothing but laugh at my own self. Like I mentioned already, I am not the guy that pity's myself. Or feels sorry for my situations in life. I do not think that gets us anywhere in life. It keeps us stagnant at the very best. Stagnant, standing in a pile of our own self - pity.

We all can dig holes for ourselves, and make horrible decisions in life. We can make complete wrecks out of our lives. And many of us were not dealt the best hand in life. I know that I was not dealt the best hand in life. Not even close. But, I was not dealt the worst either. Not even close.

If you are someone who likes to sulk, and dwell on your bad situations in life. I swear, you will fix those situations a lot faster if you thought the opposite. There are ways to retrain yourself, but they require a mental toughness that many people don't have the desire to achieve. It is sad to say that. But it is true. Laughing at your own self, is not a bad thing. Not even if you are damaging yourself in some of the worst ways. Also, other people who you know care about you, laughing at you, and trying to give you some tough love, isn't a bad thing either. Soft, weak people have a tough time with this. But the world is not going to slow down, and pity us. It will chew us up, and spit us out. And not think twice about it. Mental toughness is something that I cannot stress enough. You can never have too much of it.

So let me fill you in on this one HOT summer day at the bike trail. The day that I had my butt handed to me by my little brother.

At this time, I was already 300+ lbs. Probably even around that 320 mark. I was in denial, and still thought I could pull my athletic abilities out of my hat at any given time, if I needed them.

I used to amateur kickbox in my very early twenties. And I would do my road work, which is run, at this bike trail that goes all around the city for miles, and miles.

At the time, I was working for myself as a Mason. Which is the trade that I did for most of my life. My little brother was working with me. So he had already been in my ear about how fat and sloppy I let myself get for a while.

Well, one day, I guess I got a little "too big for my britches". And I challenged him to a long distance race at the bike trail. I think he accepted the challenge before I could even finish giving it to him.

He laughed, and laughed, and laughed, as he accepted my cocky challenge to a race of a decent distance, which I forget how long exactly now. But it was obviously way longer than I could run at that moment in time. As I am sure that you already have guessed where this story is heading?

I was probably around that 29, 30 years old age. Which would make him about 18, or 19 years old. He was 6"1, and about 150 lbs. So I was at least double his weight, and way out of any kind of shape to be trying to run a long distance. Now lets ad 100+ degree weather to the mix. Yea, I bet you are even laughing right now, am I right? It's ok! Laugh! I laughed at myself that day too. It was after I had puked out most of my dignity all over the bike trail. But, I eventually came to, and had a nice laugh at my own expense.

When we first started the race, I at least wasn't cocky enough to not run at a pace that was equal to a turtles. I basically did a power walk. And my brother stayed near me for the first few minutes, in order to get his verbal jabs in, before he darted off into the sunset. Leaving me only to eat his dust that he left behind.

He told me later that he ran to the finish line that we made for this race. And he said he waited, and waited. Wondering if I would make it to this hill where he could see me from the end.

Well, he began to actually worry, and wonder if I had passed out, or died. So he came running back in my direction to find me. I remember seeing him come running from a distance over this hill that I had not even came close to yet. I was bent over, with both hands on my knees facing his direction. Puking out every ounce of my soul all over the bike trail.

When he had seen me, I remember him stopping and just laughing hysterically as I was puking my lungs out. If I was puking, then I was not dead. So he was able to get a good laugh at my expense. Which I deserved every bit of.

Once he got his laughs finished, he ran over to me, and asked me if I was ok. I was puking out hot air by this time. We both enjoyed some good laughs, after I finally quit puking. I could not believe that I had the audacity to challenge this kid to a long distance race? What was I thinking? I still am asking myself this today.

I seriously thought that because I had ran that route, and then some, dozens, maybe even hundreds of times, when I was in great shape. That I could do it at any time, no matter what.
I was humbled that day. I could not believe how out of shape that I was. My brother had been telling me for a while, how pathetic I let myself become. He told me that when he was a little kid, he used to look up to me. And he used to have memories of me always being fixated on anything and everything sport/fitness related.

I had always been obsessed with sports, and weight training as a kid. I got my first cement weight set when I was 10 years old. I remember my grandmother buying it for me, from an ad in a penny saver magazine that I had found on my own, looking for someones old used weight set.

I started weight training with the basics, at that young age of 10 or so. I was learning how to squat, deadlift, bench press, bar dip, pull up, and more. I would read about training in magazines, and just copycat every system that I read about. I did them all.

I remember getting my other brother who is 2 years younger than me, to train with me in the back yard. He only wanted to do backarms. He was a bar dip freak as a little kid. He could pound out bar dips like a machine. Me, I would train every muscle, but I always loved squats. Which I still do to this day. Over 30 years later, and I still love squats.

Anything that was a sport, I would play it. I loved all things sport. I was that kid that had some kind of a ball in my hand at all times, bouncing it all over the place, annoying adults.

And my little brother seen that as a little kid. He seen me go from an athlete to a lush who only cared about beer :30.

My brothers tough love that he would lay on me, could easily have been taken as ridicule, and bullying. That's what soft, weak people think.

Now, do not get me wrong. If total strangers are calling you names, and constantly putting you down. That is not cool. They do not care about you. They are feeling good about tearing you down.

But when someone who cares about you does it. It might be because it is something that is needed. I needed this badly. And as stubborn of a mule that I am. I am so glad that he did not let up at any time. He could have got bored after a few days, and quit. But he was relentless. He wanted that lightbulb to finally go off in my head. And for me to reverse the damage that I was doing to myself.

I have never thanked him for that in a proper, serious way. We only talk about it from time to time, in a joking manner. This is just the way we do things. He knows though. He knows that he was the one who tipped humpty dumpty off of that wall.

And while I may have had a fall. It wasn't great enough to break me into a thousand pieces. I was able to get up, and dust myself off. And start a new journey in life.

This one day at the bike trail really pissed me off. I was pissed off at my own self. I vowed to get myself to a respectable weight again. And also wanted to get myself into the cardiovascular shape that I was once in for years of my life.

Did this happen overnight?
Absolutely not.

Did I make more mistakes on this new journey than I can count?

Absolutely.

But I have learned lessons, and am still learning lessons every day from mistakes that I make. I grow as a person from my mistakes that I make. I am barely realizing this right now! In my 40's is when I started to really see this. So this journey towards optimal health, has been a very long and bumpy road.

My Best Friend Was My Worst Enemy

You know that old saying, keep you're friends close, and you're enemies closer? Yea, well I guess I didn't quite pay attention to the true meaning of it. Because I didn't know that was exactly what I was doing for well over a decade of my life.

For many years, my best friend in the world was alcohol. I drank like clockwork, seven days a week, for years. I started drinking whatever I could in my early teens, as many people do.

And at 16, 17 years old, I would guess that I drank more than the average teen, who just gets wasted every now and then when they can get someone to give, or buy them alcohol. I would have been an everyday drinker at 16, if I had the alcohol connection to get it on a daily basis. But I did drink a lot for an underage kid. And could always drink like a grown man who had years of experience.

I am more of a natural born lush, than a drunk, or an alcoholic. Even though I suppose I am still an alcoholic. But I can steadily drink for all hours of the day, and maintain function. I can drink from morning till night regularly if I chose to. Even though I have been wasted out of my mind, several hundred times in my life. I have been in the hospital for alcohol poisoning several times. Some were worse than others.

A few of those hospital trips were after some serious drinking that would kill the average non alcoholic. If I told you how much I drank those times you would not believe me. The only people who understand drinking on that level, are the ones who can also drink on that level.

By the time I was 18, I would say that I was pretty much an everyday lush drinker. At least 90% of the days in the year I would drink, until I was 21, which for sure I was an 8 day a week lush drinker from then on, until my mid to late 30's.

At 41 now, I am still not really that many years away from drinking like a fish, each and every day. I don't really remember exactly when it was that I stopped drinking completely? But, I would guess that it has been around only 3 – 4 years or so ago, that I had my last drink. And I was tapering down my daily minimum requirement, in order to remain even keel, for a couple of years before that. But I didn't always follow my own tapering down protocol.

Will I ever drink again?

I don't know? But, I don't really want to, at least in this time in my life. I don't need it, or miss it.

Can I have just 2, or 3 beers now?

Yes, I could enjoy a couple of really good microbrews now. I love beer. And love a good high end lager, ale, IPA, stout, & more. I even made my own beer before. It was fun. I bought a kit, and would make some homebrew.

But those types of drinks were not my best friend. My best friend was cheap beer that comes in 18, and 30 packs. And hard liquors. Mostly Whiskeys, like my uncles Jack, & Jim.

I was never the belligerent drunk type. Even though of course, I have had moments. But, that is not the norm. ***I would use alcohol to maintain homeostasis.***

I could have very easily been an everyday drinker for 15 – 20 years straight! Wow. I am just doing the math in my head right now. And if I was drinking on a daily basis from 18. And I didn't stop until just a few years ago, at 38. That would be two decades.

I was still drinking regularly up until about just a handful of years ago. I think I sometimes like to act as if I wasn't. But when I think about it, I was drinking something every day. Just not anywhere near as much as I was in my 20's, and early 30's. And also a better quality of alcohol than I did in my twenties, and early to mid 30's.

I downplay my alcoholic tendencies. I always have. I am a lush by nature, and can drink from sun up to sun up! Well, maybe not right now. I would probably die if I did that now. But in my twenties, I had many of those 24+ hour drinking sessions. And many of them were all by myself. Yes, I can drink alone. Which I have heard is worse somehow? I actually prefer to drink alone.

So now that I have kind of thought of my past drinking life, right in front of your eyes here. I should probably ask myself that question again?

Will I ever have a drink or three, ever again in my life?

And the honest answer is still, I don't know?

But, I lean hard towards, I probably shouldn't, just to be on the safe side.

Like I said, I was a functioning lush, not a drunk. I was the type that could have had 20 beers in my system, and carry on a conversation with you, and you have no clue that I was legally drunk.

A typical weekday for me in my twenties was, go to work. Go to the gym after work. Maybe play some basketball at the park, or another gym after weight training, until whenever we stop, a few nights a week. Then pound my minimum beer requirements in order for me to have sweet dreams.

On nights I didn't play ball at night. I would begin my drinking immediately after the gym, as my post workout drink. Sometimes it was also my pre workout drink too. Any days off work, I could drink from the time I woke up if I wanted to. And sometimes did. Sometimes I didn't. But I always made sure to get in my alcohol requirements that my brain was telling me to, before I passed myself out.

If I was playing ball until 11 at night, and couldn't start seriously drinking until 11:30. I would just pound my beers faster, and make up for the time that I missed. I would go to sleep later if I had to. I was a Mason. So I had to wake up early in the morning. 4 am most days. If I had to stay up until 2 am to get my bodies requirements of alcohol, I would do just that. And sleep only for a couple of hours. Sleep was not important to me then.

No matter what my schedule, and life was on a particular day. I made sure that I would meet my minimum alcohol requirements before I went to sleep. I had a minimum, with no maximum. But that minimum had to be met each night.

And it wasn't necessarily a number of drinks that was my minimum. It was more about me finding my homeostasis inside of my head. So it was the alcohol levels in my bloodstream that I had to get to a certain point at minimum. This was every single day for years.

I was able to stay in both physical shape, and cardiovascular shape for many years like this too. Which is mind boggling to me now. It wasn't until I got into my later twenties, that I started to really let myself go off the edges. And like I said earlier, I was lucky to have my little brother give me that final shove off the edge, to break my own spell that I had put on myself.

When I had this fork in the road moment. And was finally going to get myself back into what I thought was good health at the time. I had NO intentions of quitting my daily drinking. NONE at ALL! That did not even cross my mind at that time. So I was going to lose 100 lbs, while still drinking like a fish each and every single day.

And guess what?

I did lose 100 lbs while still drinking like a fish each and every day! Ha!

I did not stop, or even slow down my drinking at this time. I may have even drunk more beer during this time. I could have possibly drunk less hard alcohol. But, I didn't let off of the beer gas pedal at all.

Roughly, somewhere around an 18 pack of beer, within a 3 – 4 hour window, was about the average number of beers that made me feel even keel, and normal, if I were to start drinking later in the evening. Sometimes a little less. And often times, a whole lot more! But it was rare that only a 12 pack could be enough to make me feel even keel. Maybe some IPA, with a high alcohol content per volume could do it, with only a 12 pack. That was a big maybe too, that I often didn't allow to be found out. Because I always had alcohol on deck, just in case those situations arose. Hard liquor was always my ace in the hole, if I really needed it.

Like I said, it was about the alcohol in my bloodstream, over the number of beers I drank. And if I was drinking all day, I would just maintain my homeostasis by continually drinking like clockwork. I am not proud of this. I am not embarrassed either. I just need to make sure that I never become that person who relies on alcohol again.

When I finally decided that enough was enough, as far as being a fat 320 lbs goes. I kicked myself in the butt immediately, and did the only thing I really ever knew how to do then. And that was WORK. One thing that I am proud of, is my work ethic. I have the ability to work myself to the bone, which isn't healthy. I know this now. But all that I really knew then was that hard work always pays off. And in general it does.

But, there are always limits to how hard we should work, before we are going the other way, and damaging our bodies.

I made so many mistakes in this process of losing the initial 90 lbs in 90 days. I went from 320 lbs, to 230 lbs, in just 90 days. That I remember doing, and completing my mission. I made a bet with my little brother that I could do it. He knew I could do it too. He just had to motivate me by telling me that I was going to give up. If I did not have him motivating me in that way, I may have very well gave up early. So we made a bet. And I showed him pictures of my weight on the scale the entire time I was dropping the weight.

I had always kind of thought that I knew at least the basics of nutrition at this time. Because I was into athletics, and weight training. I followed all kinds of diets that were in the muscle magazines for years, and thought that was how healthy people eat. I would still eat so much processed foods, from fast foods, microwaveable foods, junk foods, and of course beer.

My caloric intake from beer a day was probably more than many people consume from their food in a day. My calories had to be insanely high. Which if they were from the proper sources, wouldn't have been so bad. I worked in a brutal trade, in high heats in the summer time. And I lived a very high fuel burning lifestyle outside of my job as well.

So I required really high calories to live. But the sources of my calories were from mostly processed crap. Man made garbage. I changed none of this during this initial weight loss. I "made up for it", with extreme volume cardio. And I mean a ton of cardio!

This was one of my many mistakes I made!

But I would not change it for the world. I learned from every single mistake that I made. And am here to share my mistakes with you, so you do not possibly make the same ones. At this time my thinking was that if I try and punch a hole in a block wall, it does not make a hole. That means that I obviously didn't punch it hard enough. And I must punch it harder next time to make a hole.

I was a stupid Neanderthal.

I took myself from fat & lazy slob who gave up on myself. To a cardio freak instantly, from day 1. I went balls to the walls with the cardio, and was dead set on losing a specific amount of bodyweight, no matter what. Even though I could have made life so much easier on myself had I knew about nutrition then, as much as I do now.

If I Knew Then What I Know Now

If I only knew then, what I know now about nutrition alone. I would have had such a healthier weight loss experience. It is a good thing that I was young, already previously in great shape at times in my life. And also I do have good genetics, and am not prone to sickness, and diseases(knock on wood). Like I said, I can work like a slave. Nose to the grindstone is all that I ever knew.

I did not run any bloodwork on myself either. Which is something that if I could go back and do all over again, I would have got bloodwork done on myself before, during, and after this big weight loss. I imagine my bloodwork being horrible at this time. Good genetics can only hold on for so long before they become defeated by a toxic lifestyle.

So what exactly would I have done differently if I knew then what I know now?

Let's begin with the most important aspect. And that is nutrition. Our nutrition SHOULD BE the most important aspect of our lives, each and every day, until we kick the bucket. PERIOD. This is not debatable. How many people put their own nutritional needs first in their lives? Very few. In our western culture, it is next to none.

Even people who accidently stay moderately healthy, due to genetics, age, and non addictive personalities, still more than likely don't put their nutritional needs first in their lives. I know that I sure didn't for most of my life. I didn't learn this until I was in my mid 30's, and really trying to learn about my own body, and what can make me thrive longer on this planet.

I talk about this all the time. There are too many distractions. We are losing our archaic instincts of survival. It is not going to get better either, as technology is leading us down this path. The better the technology gets, the dumber we all seem to get. Even though we think that we are getting smarter, because we have got so much information at our fingertips.

What is the radius of Jupiter in meters?

I know!!!!!!

69.911 million meters.

I just googled it in 2 seconds. Now I am a genius!

You see, we think we know everything because we can be told things on the internet in a blink of an eye. But who figured that equation out? Is it even accurate? Did someone just completely guess that, and now it is so?

Now obviously, scientists who are light years smarter than we are, figured those numbers out. And I will sleep easy tonight, believing them to be accurate. But I hope you get the point that I am making here?

Just because we can google anything that we want, and find the answer to it in less than a few seconds. That does not mean that we are now as smart as the geeks who actually know how to figure that all out, with a shoe box with a tiny little hole in it, and a pad and pencil.

The internet is great. I make my living on it. I love it. And learning is great. Even entertainment is great. We all need that. But they all should have their place in our lives, so they do not become distractions to us. There is a such thing as information overload. I have had it so many times in my life. Especially since I began to make my living providing information, and entertainment to other people via the internet. I have had many times when I needed to back away, and let the information ooze from my ears, so that I can think clearly.

To get back to the topic of nutrition. This is something that at this time in my life, I didn't really dwell on. I always had thought that if I just followed what was in magazines, or what was popular, I would be eating healthy by default. This was pre internet era. The internet in the last 4, or 5 years has really boomed.

The internet today, and the amount of information out there in health & nutrition, is enough to be a distraction for most people. Especially people who know nothing to very little about their own nutrition. And that is almost everyone. They just don't know that, because they can google everything, and know everything about everything.

A part of me is kind of glad that I wasn't really searching all over the web at this time in my life, for information on nutrition. And in 2006, the information on the web was not what it is in 2018. We are in manic times. Everyone is fighting for you're business. What makes it to the top of the lists, and in front of the masses eyes, is always based on marketing. Valuable, factual information is not really as important as marketability. So do not just believe what you read, see, or hear. You must figure these things out on your own.

In 2013, I wrote some books, that in them I was telling people that all of the fad diets at that time, were stemmed from basic bodybuilding types of diets. And they were, and still are. This isn't the worst thing in the world. As even a basic bodybuilding rice, chicken, and broccoli type of diet is far better than fast food. But nutrition for optimal health, and even taking it further than that, requires a dedication to becoming in tune with ones own body, from the inside out. This doesn't happen overnight. And requires an obsession with what is important.

It all begins with consuming 100% unprocessed foods.

That is the base to start from. I was saying this in 2013, and I still say it to this day. I was learning this sometime around 2008, or 9ish. Which is a few years after my, I have had enough of myself moment on that bike trail. I had already lost 100 lbs, and kept it off, with continued hard work. I still work hard. I will always work hard. I am not trying to say to avoid hard work. Life is hard. Hard work is a good thing. And needed to lose a massive amount of weight, and keep it off for life.

But around this 2008, 09, time, is when I really started to desire to learn about my own nutritional needs. And I now have a burning desire to never stop learning about them. I wrote a song many years ago, called How Addiction Turns Into Obsession. I like to use this song title now, in explaining how deep my obsession goes with my own personal vitality. It is way beyond and addiction. I am an addict. It runs through my veins at all times. I may as well channel it towards something that is pure, and makes me become a better me. So a handful of years ago, I chose to become addicted to my longevity. And find a way to be ok with living my own self. I still have trouble with that second one. And I probably always will. But hopefully I have got many years left on this earth to figure it out.

Unprocessed Foods vs Processed Foods

Everybody knows all about this right?

I mean, we can all google it in two seconds. Most of us don't even have to google anything. We know the difference between processed and unprocessed foods. Because we know everything about everything, right? Well then, how come we don't apply any of this knowledge that we have? Because unprocessed foods are what leads us in the right direction towards optimal health. Do we not want optimal health? We sure act like we don't if we consume any amount of processed foods in our diet.

In 2006, I knew the difference between processed foods and unprocessed foods. Asking me if I did may have even been an insult to my intelligence. Did I really know the difference? Or did I know the googling version of the difference?

Yea, I didn't know **jack s**t!**

I am still learning the differences between processed and unprocessed calories. And the effects both have on our bodies. I will never stop learning about this subject. Because there is so much information to process, without getting that dreaded information overload syndrome.

So had I known then, what I know now. I would have obviously put myself on a similar diet, and training program that I am doing right now. This is because I have finally perfected both to fit my own personal needs. And by perfected, I mean as close to perfected as I have ever gotten it to date. There is always room for more improvements. But right now, I am in the best health of my life. With blood work to prove that. My health age is that of a teenager. My testosterone is around 1000, at 41 years of age, with NO TRT, HRT, or shooting up steroids, and acting like I don't. You know, kind of like many of the leaders in health & fitness on the internet do. Yea, they won't show their blood work. There is a lot of things they don't want you to see, that's why. I posted my recent blood work on my new YouTube Channel – Dexter the vEGGan.

So let me be personal trainer, and nutritional advisor to my old 320 lb self. And let you know exactly what I would have had myself do both with nutrition, and training, in order to lose that 90 lbs in 90 days, that I initially lost, and won that bet with my brother by the way. Lets not forget that. I won!

I actually made some other bets with him later too. Like getting myself under 200 lbs. Which even I didn't think I would ever get down to at that time. Once I got to around 230 lbs, it was a different type of weight loss journey than before. A much harder one in some ways to be honest.

But I did stay around 230 lbs for a while. And even floated up close to 240. But, I never let myself go past that ever again. I made sure that I was not going to let myself float back up in weight. I even began to reverse my thinking into wanting to be as small as possible, instead of wanting to be a mass monster, like I wanted to be since a small child. They call this Bigorexia now. A term that I actually only recently learned in the last handful of years from the internet. Ha!

I had, and can always have this Bigorexia thing(not sure if I should call it a disease). I naturally hate my body. And have always thought that I was extra small. Even when I was well over 200 lbs. I could be 240 lbs, and very big, and lean for a guy not on steroids. And I would look in the mirror and be disgusted with my puny little biceps. If I did steroids at that time, I would have easily had those biceps that I wanted. The biceps that you can only get by doing steroids. I actually had traps of a steroid user. But that was my genetics. My legs were huge too. But my arms were always the smallest thing, that I could never make grow how I wanted them too. I wanted them to look like a roiders arms.

Do me a favor, and go and watch many of my videos. I have thousands of social media videos of myself doing various things. Do you ever see me in a short sleeve shirt? The answer is no.

And you never will. I never will either. I will wear long sleeve shirts for the rest of my life. Just so that way I don't ever fall back into that mindset. It sounds childish. And it is childish. But it is real. If I wore short sleeve shirts, I would have a constant feeling crawling down my spine, similar to a cat scratching a chalkboard. This would be how I would feel inside. So my band aid is long sleeve shirts. And you know what? I am really good with that. I like how I dress anyways. I am the only person who dresses like me on the planet. And I do that on purpose. This is just my personality. So the long sleeve shirt under the short sleeve shirt thing, is something that I like to do anyways. But, that is what I will tell people in public who ask me about the way I dress. I am letting you know now, one of my many little secrets.

Remember, I am completely fine with this. I do not dwell on something as minute as this. I never think about it. I just made it a habit. And it became part of who I am. Sometimes this can be better than making an ordeal out of every single thing. I am a grown man. I can figure out a way to not look at my arms, and think of how small and spaghetti – like they are. Thank you Lou Ferrigno for the "spaghetti arms" memes.

My nutrition & training protocol I would give to my old 320 lb self:

Nutrition:
Oh my God, where to begin? I would give my old self a complete overhaul of my diet. Now, let's just pretend that I would have listened to my current self. Which I wouldn't have. But, let's pretend that I did. At least when it came to alcohol. I was not ready to give that up, for several years after even.

Lets say that I hopped into my 1985 Delorean, and traveled back in time, to good old 2006. And had a one on one, heart to heart talk with my 29 year old self. Just as I was about to embark on this new 90 lbs, in 90 days weight loss bet that had made with my little brother.

If I would have listened to 2018 me, and cut out alcohol, just by itself. I would have eliminated close to, and even over 2,000 calories a day, just from beer! Depending on the type of beer I was drinking. I was drinking at least very close to 2000 calories each day, if I drank light beer that day. And well over 2000 calories if I was drinking anything else. And that is if I just drank an 18 pack, of light beer. Who does that? Little girls?

So my guess is that most days I was consuming over 2000 calories from beer. That is insane. And that was for well over a decade. And probably closer to a decade and a half, if I were to be honest about it. Can you see why I knock on wood when I mention my decent genetics? I am blessed to not have any long term side effects, or liver, or kidney issues.

If I were to just cut out the alcohol calories alone, I would have probably lost 20 lbs pretty quickly, from water weight. I would not even have to do any exercise at all to lose the initial water weight from cutting out the alcohol.

Before I would start figuring out a diet for my old self. I would make my old self get a full panel blood test drawn. And find out what deficiencies I had. And I imagine that I had plenty of nutrient deficiencies. I would somewhat base my food selection on that, even though my food selection is natural unprocessed foods, that are going to provide all of the nutrition needed for my body, daily. But, it is always good to know what you are lacking, and deficient in.

Vitamin D3:

If I knew about vitamin d3 then, oh man, I would have been down the road to optimal health a lot sooner. I have made such an effort to get my vitamin d up to 100 ng/ml. And I will keep it there too.

There is a correlation between my vitamin d, and my testosterone. When my vitamin d is up. So are my test levels. I am someone who thrives off of the sun. I always have, even before I ever knew the suns relation to vitamin d. I feel like superman if I can get at least an hour of sun exposure on 75% of my body a day. And this is every day. And if I can get two hours, that makes me feel even more superhuman.

This is only because of the diet that I currently eat. Which allows my body to absorb the benefits of the sun fully, and not be damaging to my body. When I cannot get as much sun exposure as I really want. I then supplement vitamin d3. But for me, the sun exposure on most of my body, is really what I thrive on. It's like plugging me into a socket, and charging up my battery for the day.

If we are healthy enough, our body will react this way to the sun. It is our battery charger in the sky. If we are unhealthy, then we can tend to reject the benefits from the powerful sun. And that is when it can do more damage to us than good.

Everyone is different. Also skin tone plays a big role in how much sun each individual can require, and tolerate. But for me, sun is my battery charger. I need it daily.

I worked outdoors my entire life. And in extreme heats, in the blazing sun. But that is not the same. When you work outside in the sun, if you are smart, you cover up your body. Some people have their forearms showing, by wearing short sleeves. But this is not enough skin exposure to really get the full benefits of sun exposure to the skin. You really need to be 75% unclothed. At least 50%. You wont get a sufficient amount of sun exposure just working outdoors with your clothes on. And some people think you just need your eyes to see sun for 30 minutes a day. I have no clue where they hear this from, but this is also not good enough.

So I would have convinced my old self of the benefits of the hormone vitamin d. And I would have made myself go out of my way to get several hours a week of sun exposure on at least half of my body. I would have taken a vitamin d3 supplement as well. 2,000 – 5,000 IU's a day. I was working outdoors at the time, in a pretty brutal masonry trade. So my desire to get more sun, after being in the sun all day, wouldn't have been strong. Even though I always loved sun, even before this. I just didn't know the importance of vitamin d, and sun exposure on my body. So my vitamin d levels would have been very important to me. And supplementing would be something that I would have done, along with getting full body sun exposure.

What would I eat?

I remember going on this Subway binge at this time. Hey, Jarod did it. And he lost a lot more weight than I did. I did do a lot of Subway during this weight loss. Which isn't the most horrible thing in the world. Not even close to optimal. But better than what a lot of people eat on a regular basis.

My caloric intake at this time had to be really high. But not as high as it may seem. Beer was like food to me. I did not eat while I drank. I ate before, and hopefully after. When I drank on days that I worked the next day, it was hopefully about just getting myself to even keel. Then eating right before passing out. I say hopefully, because sometimes, I would go past that point, and just drink myself to sleep. But ideally, I liked to always eat something, just before I slept.

I ate everything. I didn't really have unprocessed vs processed foods on my mind during those years. Although, I often would follow standard bodybuilding chicken, rice, and a little veggies diets. Not the worst thing in the world, as long as you aren't smothering it with condiments. But when I was at my worst, I really ate horribly. Lots of processed junk. Frozen dinner meals. Fast food, and a lot of pizza. Basically, the standard American diet. Although, I was never really a candy eater. But, my alcohol was my candy. So I was making up for that with beer.

I barbequed a lot. And always ate a ton of meat. Meat, meat and more meat, was what I thought was good for being big and strong. I had a high protein mentality for many years. It was hard to let go of my high protein mentality when I decided to eliminate meat, and also dairy from my life, sometime around 2009, 10ish. After I watched the documentary Earthlings. It changed my life, for the better, eventually.

So because I was not at the time of my life yet when I was weening myself off of dairy, and meat. I will just allow myself one of those things. And that is the meat. I would have made myself get off all dairy day one. If I could not do that. I would have gave myself a small amount of dairy from either plain cottage cheese, or plain greek yogurt. But a very small amount. And plain isn't really good tasting. So I may have not even touched it then.

I would have given myself an easy to follow meal plan that was compatible with my job. I would love to say to my old self, eat exactly like I eat now in 2018. But that is not compatible with the job of a mason. At least not the order the meals are eaten in.

I would have taught my old self, just how basic, and easy food is, and should be. The calories are our energy. Our fuel. Unprocessed fuel is what we run best on. Now how do we figure out which calories our bodies run best on?

Calories:

- **Protein - 4 calories per gram**
- **Carbohydrate - 4 calories per gram**
- **Fat – 9 calories per gram**
- **Alcohol – 7 calories per gram**

Remember what I said earlier in this book about distractions? Well, dwelling on these bullet points above, can be a distraction for many. And the internet today tends to make people dwell on these bullet points way too much.

Unprocessed foods balance out everything.

My old self was basically fixated on one of those bullet points. And that one is the protein. Which, not to downplay it at all, because protein is important. But it might be the least important of the four macronutrients we can get our energy (calories) from.

Why?

Because if we eliminate the fourth one (the alcohol). And Give our body what 2, and 3 needs. The first one (protein) will fall right into place. Diet is so easy. We just need to not let the distractions of hype, and excellent marketing tactics, sway us from believing that. I would have told my old self that micronutrient absorption is what our body desires. How do we get the best absorption of micronutrients? We get this from consuming real, whole foods. Unprocessed foods.

The best quality micronutrients, are in the best quality macronutrients. This makes sense right? This is what we should be fueling our bodies with. The best quality of macronutrients (calories, energy). In order for our bodies to absorb the high quality micronutrients, that all of our cells, and organs are begging for.

When it comes to the macronutrients, I would quickly tell my old self...

- Protein – think muscle.
- Fat – think hormones.
- Carbs – think LIFE!
- Alcohol – Think DEATH!

See how simple that is? Anyone can understand that. So I would not even focus on my old self's caloric intake just yet. Because if I got my old self to listen to me up to this point. The foods I would be now consuming would pretty much fix that caloric overdose by default.

Of course, if I quit drinking cold Turkey, would I have alcohol withdrawls? Oh yes, I would. But I also was the one who did that to myself. I would need to own up to that, and deal with the consequences. Like I said, the loss in calories from beer alone would have dropped a lot of water weight off of my body. I would not have really wanted to drop 2000 more calories from the food at the same time. So the diet would have to taper down to a perfect caloric intake.

I was going nuts with the intense cardio, which I will get into my training in a bit. Plus with my job being a very physical trade, and in the summer high heats. I burned through a lot more calories than the average couch potato.

I would have had to make up for some of those beer calories with real food. Or my energy levels would have tanked.

So if I were to eliminate the alcohol in one fell swoop. I would have to taper down the total calories, instead of just dropping several thousand calories a day immediately.

So what would be the best fix for that?

LIFE!

AKA – Fruit.

Yes, contrary to what half of the internet (distractions) are constantly trying to tell us. Fruit is in fact not just good for us. But, it is the best source of carbohydrate that we can consume. If we seek out the highest quality micronutrients for our body. Then fruit is the ultimate place to find them. And, for some weird reason, fruit also contains high quality macronutrients. Hmmm. Go figure, huh? Fruit = life.

So I would tell my old self that fruit was unlimited. Eat as much of it as I want, and whenever I want it. If I needed to get myself addicted to fruit, to make up for the addiction to alcohol, so be it. Instead of drinking an 18 pack of beer. Eat 18 bananas. Which addiction do you think is the better choice?

Here is kind of a basic way that I would line my old self out to eat each day, from morning until night.

In the morning, I would have myself eat oats, and mixed berries. They can be cooked in water only, or raw. And I would not put a quantity limit on this meal. Just eat until I was full. I would also add in a couple of bananas, or more if I wanted more than 2.

Working in construction, and being as active as I was, my water intake was always crazy high, as needed. So I would not need to remind myself about water intake. I would have told myself to not drink tap water though. But, you do what you got to do.

Electrolytes:

To me back then, electrolytes meant Gatorade. I think to most people electrolytes means some kind of sports drink. I would make sure that I had my old self's electrolytes on point. This is so important, especially for really active people, as I was. Potassium especially, is something many people are always deficient in.

And this always surprises people, but so is sodium. Sodium, like good carbohydrates, and fructose from fruits, is not the devil. The low sodium distraction is not something that most people should listen to, and follow. Hey, even I got caught up in it before. I tried to reduce sodium from my diet at one time in my life, by constantly checking labels on my food, and only buying low sodium PROCESSED FOODS! I was distracted by the information overload being put on me, by whatever fad it was that I got lured into.

If a person is eating mostly unprocessed foods even. They will still probably need to add sodium into their diet to reach the minimum recommended amount. Which I need even more than the minimum recommended amount. And so does everyone else who is very active. And if you eat completely 100% unprocessed foods. You will need to add sodium into each meal, in order to reach that daily recommended minimum.

So if I were taking my old self off of processed foods. Knowing the activity level that I lived daily. I would make sure that I added good salt (iodized salt most meals) with each and every meal that I consumed. My goal would be to get at least 4500 mg a day of sodium. Adding some good quality salt to everything I eat, to taste, does that. So there would be no need to measure it all out. Just add it to taste, in every single meal.

I would be shooting for 5400 mg of potassium, which is not easy to achieve without eating the right foods, moderate to high in potassium.

Most people are potassium deficient. I once read an article online by a Doctor, who said that everyone is potassium deficient. Well Doc. I'm not. And in order for me to not be potassium deficient. I need to eat certain types of foods each day, or I can even come up short of my personal 5400 mg daily requirements. **3500 – 4700 is what the FDA recommends.**

All of the electrolytes, besides sodium, I would be able to consume my requirements with food. If I focus on getting my potassium in, the rest all balance themselves out in those food choices that I make. Learning every single detail, to every single micronutrient that we need to run on high idle, is fine. But, it is not always necessary. I would not want to overload my old self with information. I would just tell my old self to figure out what types of foods are moderate, and high in potassium. And to start paying attention to my potassium, and sodium intake. I would have myself count the mg until I was able to get my requirements by just eating on instinct. It won't take long before that happens.

With just the unlimited amount of fruit I would be eating alone, I could get my potassium requirements. But I would also add in foods like tubers, beans, & lots of greens, which all contain good amounts of potassium. I would exceed my requirements if I ate the proper foods each day. If I started this day one, I would immediately feel some good effects from this.

Rice cooker:

I have been telling people to get a rice cooker for years now. I am the self - proclaimed King of rice cooking.

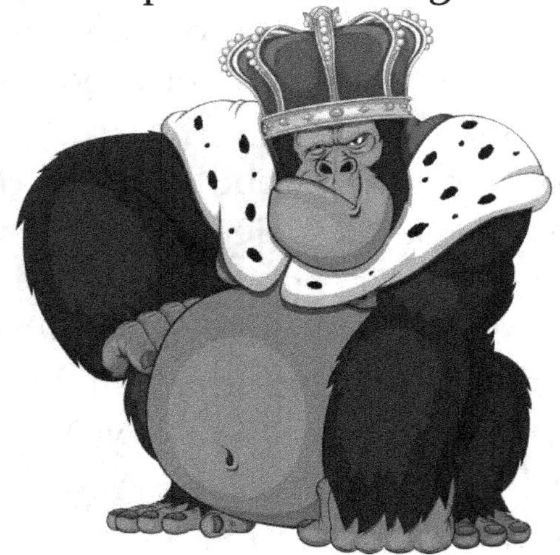

I would have went back in time to visit my old self, carrying a rice cooker in my hands as a gift of peace. Possibly a blender as well. But for sure a rice cooker. This is what I would have my old self cook most of my food in. And not just for the convenience of it either. But also because a rice cooker actually helps a person eat healthier, even when they are really trying to eat healthier.

Cooking in a rice cooker, gives you pretty much only healthy choices of foods to cook with. At least what you put inside of the rice cooker. And you don't need to cook anything in oils, butter, or anything other than water.

I would have my old self cook rice cooker meals (rice cooker meatless goulashes as I call them) in bulk. Fill the thing up, and eat off of it until it's empty. Then continue the cycle for life.

The cooking possibilities in a rice cooker are endless. These are the staple foods that I would have my old self consume on a regular basis. I would give my old self a lot of room to pick and choose any combination of all of these foods. Because they all are good choices, no matter how you mix them together.

- **All rices – white, brown, wild.**
- **All quinoas – every color that exists.**
- **All lentils – every color.**
- **All tubers – sweet, red, golden, russet, yams, everything that is a tuber is open season.**

These are the basic main carb choices I would choose from. I could mix and match any, and all of them as I desired. There are endless ways to mix all of these types of foods together in a rice cooker. Along with carbs from fruit. These would be my staple calories. Taking a close second to the fruit calories, which would be the majority of my calories in a day.

I would also tell my old self to mix fruits inside of the rice cooker with these foods. Many fruits can be cooked inside of the rice cooker along with the foods I mentioned above. Some of my favorites are:

- **Pineapple – frozen**
- **Raisins**
- **Dates**
- **Mango – frozen**
- **Blueberries – frozen**
- **Honey crisp apples – or any other apple.**

There are more, but these are just a few of my favorite fruits that I like to mix into my rice cooker with my meatless goulashes. I will get to the meat in a bit.

So we have got plenty of carb staples, along with fruits to mix together into the rice cooker. Now, we need to get some vegetables in it, and close the lid, and click start.

All vegetables are open season. And this can be cooked, or raw. I would tell my old self to make sure and get a mix of veggies inside of each of these rice cooker goulashes. I would tell myself that a lot of garlic, and all flavors of onion are a must. Each cooked meal. And maybe even dice the onions, and add them on top raw. The garlic can be cooked inside of the rice cooker. I would work myself up to a bulb a day. Not just a clove or two, but an entire bulb.

Some good vegetable choices I would give myself to cook inside of the rice cooker are:

- **Frozen or raw spinach**
- **Frozen or raw kale**
- **Frozen peas**
- **Frozen or raw squashes**
- **Frozen or raw greenbeans**
- **Frozen or raw carrots**

These are all easily accessible, and cheap to buy. And if eaten daily, along with all of the other natural foods, provides the micronutrients our body desires to run at its best. A lot of the micronutrients are going to come from fruits. As they should be. But a wide range of vegetables would be mixed into my cooked meals daily.

And how many cooked meals would I be eating a day?

Well, first, with my schedule, I would be cooking these meatless goulashes at night, and preparing them for the next day. Or just leaving it in the cooker, and putting it in the refrigerator until I got up in the morning and prepared my lunch for the day. If I didn't have to work out in a filthy, hot, blow and go trade. Ideally, I would only have myself eat 1, or 2 cooked meals. And all at night. I would have my old self eat an entire watermelon for my second meal, if the circumstances allowed this to happen.

And they didn't. It is too hard to take a watermelon to a job like that. And you are pretty filthy dirty each day. The whole scenario won't really allow that to happen. If I was working from my own home, indoors. And could pee whenever I needed to. I would definitely have my old self eat an entire watermelon (minimum) a day if possible. If there are no watermelons available. Mix more fruits into the diet for the second meal.

But in this case, I would have myself take however much of my goulash that felt I needed to eat that day. Along with some bananas, and extra salt. This would be an easy to prepare, and easy to digest choice, as I worked during the day.

If I needed some extra fats:

If I ever felt like my body needed some extra fats in the day. I would tell my old self to either add an avocado to my cooked meal. Or I would give myself 1 – 2 tablespoons of natural peanut butter. But no more. And this shouldn't be daily really. Just some days those extra calories from good fats are really good to consume. If anything, for satiation purposes.

I would go to the gym after work. So my pre workout meal, would be fruit & oats. Whatever I wanted. There is nothing complicated about this. Fruit could actually be my pre & post workout food if I felt like I needed it. And I would not add any caffeine or stimulant into the pre workout meals.

So we come to after the gym. When I would typically start pounding the beers down. And remember, I drank beer all through this weight loss. I drank exactly the same as I always did. I drank beer, and sunk into my guitar often times.

But since we are make believing that I quit drinking all together. I would have had myself eat for sure 1, or 2 (if I was having calorie/hunger withdrawls) cooked meals before I went to sleep. I would never put a daily calorie limit on myself. Especially at this time. I would however have my old self count not just my total calories. But count the carbs, protein, and fat grams and calories, as best as I could. And I am sure I would be off on my count. But, it is good to get a close idea of where you are at, calorie-wise. So I would be logging all of this down daily. At least until it all became instinctive to me.

My calories from fruit would be well over 1000 on a work day. And maybe even up to 2000 calories a day. Pretty much replacing those beer calories. I like my fruit calories to be more than half of my total calories in a day. At this time, I would like my fruit calories to be even more of my total calories. Even up to 75%. If I didn't have to work in the trade I worked in, I could do that. But, I would have more than likely been around 50 – 60% calories from fruit. That is still great. I would feel the effects of this pretty quickly. Even if I was still craving the alcohol. My body would be drenched in micronutrients that it needed.

Meat, protein, & fats

At night is where I would give myself just one animal protein meal, to go along with the rice cooker meatless goulashes that I would be continually making. If I ate a cooked meal in the day, it would all be plant based. No animal products until night time. I was still eating all things meat back then. So let's just say that I allowed myself to continue to eat meats.

I would allow just one meal to have some meat, or animal product in it. But I would do it like this:

- **Day 1 – 4 – 8 oz of grass fed Bison.**
- **Day 2 – 4 – 6 whole eggs, pasture raised.**
- **Day 3 – 4 – 8 oz of wild caught Salmon with skin.**
- **Day 4 – 4 – 6 whole eggs, pasture raised.**
- **Day 5 – 4 – 8 oz of grass fed Bison.**
- **Day 6 – 4 – 6 whole eggs, pasture raised.**
- **Day 7 – 4 – 8 oz of wild caught Salmon with skin.**
- *** Replace one of those days with oysters, or other shellfish if desired.**

That's it for the animal products for the week. And I would have myself cook these products in no oils, or butters. It doesn't matter how I cooked them. Just not in any other fats, or processed oils.

That is just an average of 25 – 50 grams of protein from animal products a day. My jaw would have been literally dropped to the floor at this time. How was I going to be a man, and eat only 25 – 50 grams of protein a day from animal products? Surely this must be a mistake, I would ask my future self? Don't you mean for each meal?

No! A day...

For now!

After a while, I would convince my old self to start having some plant based days, without any animal products mixed into the week. 1, or 2 a week.

This is pretty much it for the nutrition side. I would put my old self on a non processed foods lifestyle. And have myself eventually become an instinctive eater. It takes a little while. But it is worth it.

When in doubt? Eat Fruit.

Fruit would be the center of my universe. With all of the intense cardio that I put myself through to lose this initial 90 lbs. I really would have had more energy. And recovered better, had I made a wide variety of fruits (especially watermelon) the bigger percentage of my overall caloric intake.

Training:

I remember that last day in the bet I had made with my brother. I was a little over 230 lbs. And I needed to burn off some water weight to go below it, so I could text my brother a picture of the scale at the gym showing under 230. The last 20, 30 lbs were the really tough ones to get off. The first 20, or 30 lbs, were somewhat the easiest to lose. But, I was the most out of shape at that weight.

So, physically, they were not easy pounds to lose. At 250 lbs, I was looking like I was strong, and explosive. Even though I was not really. Because I was fixated on losing a specific number of pounds. And my focus was on cardio. A lot of cardio, and sauna. To lose those last pounds to win the bet, I spent several hours at the gym, back and forth from the sauna to the stair master. I was cutting weight as if I had a weigh in for a fight. I bundled up in layers of clothes, and just grinded it out.

It is not the smartest weight cutting method in the world. But, I was young, and I have worked harder than that for sport before. I just mimicked the only way that I knew how to cut weight. By sweating it out of me. It does work. And a sauna is great for us. Just not hours of it at a time. I probably did about 4 hours of cardio, sauna, cardio, sauna, that last day. And the days before it, I was warming myself up for it, knowing that I would need it.

If I had to do it over again, I still would keep a good amount of cardio in. Just not as much. And not as high of intensity as I did it. I kept my cardio on machines. Which is a good thing at high weights. You don't want to be running, or jumping around on hard floor at heavy weights. It just isn't good for the joints. So I would keep all of the cardio machine work I did in, at less intensity.

I love cardio machines. All of them. Once again, the internet sometimes comes in and tries to lure us into the latest fad workout, by putting down cardio machines. This is popular right now. Being anti cardio machine. Well, it's just another distraction. Cardio machines are fine.

I just got off of one not more than a half an hour ago. After training, I walked on a treadmill at 4.0 incline, 3.4 speed for over a half an hour. Treadmill cardio for me, is for my brain more than anything. I think about all kinds of things. I thought about this book that I am currently writing, amongst many other things during this nice little brisk walk on a treadmill. Now, I am back home, eating the rest of a watermelon that I cut up before the gym, typing this out. Trying not to get watermelon juice all over my keypad. These days, I actually prefer lower intensity cardio, such as what I did today. You don't have to go balls out in order to make progress. In fact, most people should never go balls out period.

My higher intensity cardio was done on a stair stepper, and a stationary bike. Both of them can be done at intensities all over the map. I would make up workouts, and little mini goals that I would give myself to complete on the spot. I just made the cardio a game that I played with myself. I still do this all the time on those machines.

I like to ride the stationary bike with my butt off the seat. So I just come up with little challenges, and games, based on what I am feeling like that particular moment. I adjust the levels of difficulty however I feel like. It doesn't have to be anything more than that. People overcomplicate things way too much. Movement of any kind, is better than no movement at all.

I did and still do the same thing on the stair stepper. I would skip steps, raise and lower the speeds, step from my toes only. Wear weighted vests, ankle weights, and not touch the machine with my hands. I personally don't and never have done any of that sideways, and backwards stepping like I see girls do all the time. I just did everything with myself facing forward. And I still do those things on stair steppers from time to time. If I am doing a stair stepper or a stationary bike. You can bet on it that I am playing some kind of internal game with myself, in order to make myself not think about anything at all. Which sometimes, not thinking is good too. The treadmill walks are for my thinking of things in life.

What I did do, that I wish I didn't do, was that I didn't get back into weight training during this weight loss. I basically quit training weights for a while, during this time in my life that I let myself go. I don't really remember how long it was. But it was long enough. Probably over a year. Maybe 2 years even. I may have occasionally popped into the gym every now and then. But my training motivation was not there.

When I decided to lose this 90 lbs in 90 days. I did it without weight training. I may have done a little machine fluff. But I didn't do any of the basic movements that I had done my whole life. I really wish that I did.

The diet is the most important thing when it comes to weight loss. I was not going to stop drinking like a fish. So I over compensated with hours of medium to high intensity cardio. That is really dumb. But, I was stubborn.

So if I were to get my old self on this unprocessed foods diet. I would have made sure that I kept in squats at least. I would have added in pull ups, dips, and pushups too. Just basic movements. Pull ups would have been difficult at 320 lbs. I imagine I would have been doing them assisted. Which is good for the ego. Heck, I may have even been doing dips assisted as well. But squats would have been beneficial, and should have been a staple of my training.

I also would have introduced my old self to the pre training workout that I do now, which is what keeps me **Agile – Mobile – Virile.**

These are my 3 – iles that I live by, and base my focus on. My goal is to be as agile, mobile, and virile, as I possibly can for life. This 20 – 30 minute pre training workout that I have done for several years now, is the most important half hour of my day. I would have to adjust some of the movements, and stretches to fit my old 300 lb self's level. But I would make sure that I began doing these series of movements, and stretches, from then on out.

The training doesn't matter nearly as much as the diet, when it comes to a weight loss such as this. I would really have benefitted at this time from the nutritional knowledge that I have learned over the years. Through so much trial and error, I have found the fountain of youth diet, for myself, if there is such a thing. I believe that there is. I am living it right now. I am consistently getting younger, as I age in years. Some people may laugh, but I am proving this to be possible. Our minds are very powerful. The brain has abilities that even our own brains cannot comprehend. Taking mind over matter, and turning it into **MIND OVER MATTER, &** staying consistent with applying it 25/8/366. If there is one thing that I really want you to get from reading this book it is...

Consistency

Yes, consistency is the key to making all things possible, that may seem impossible. A tiny drip of water can drill a hole in a boulder, if it is consistently dripping in the same exact spot.

Hey, there is one more thing we can google and find the answer to I bet? Let's race to google and see who becomes the genius first? I will let you win this one. You can tell me how long a drip of water has to drip onto a rock before it begins to create a hole? I will believe you to be Einstein.

When it came down to me losing initially 90 lbs in 90 days. Then, going down under 230 lbs to 220 lbs. Then, going down under 220 lbs to 210 lbs. Then, going down under 210 lbs to 200 lbs. Then, going down again under 200 lbs, to 190 lbs, and even sometimes playing around in the 180's for the fun of it. This was all accomplished by my consistency. Yea, I am a little crazy too. But consistency is what made that scale drop down, and down, and down each day. And the scale doesn't even matter. I was trying to win a bet. But, the goal of becoming healthy once again, is what matters most. But what good is becoming healthy once again, if you don't not just stay healthy. Let's take this further than that. What good is getting sick of being a fat mess, and motivating myself to become healthy, if I don't continue to motivate myself to become healthier, each and every day.

This is where I am at right now, at this point in my life. And I have been there for several years now. My mind has been there. Some of my actions in the beginning may not have shown that my mind was there. But life tends to enjoy throwing sticks into our spokes, and watching us eat it all over the concrete.

2010ish was when I think that I really began to think about my longevity, and vitality seriously. Like really seriously. I made so many mistakes in trying to find the perfect way of eating. So many. I would not change those mistakes either. I am where I am at today in my nutrition because of those mistakes. And many of them were not really huge mistakes either.

Like going 100% plant based vegan in 2015, for 1 year. I did it as good as it can be done. I was limiting my processed foods before this, and really made sure that I consumed a 90+% unprocessed food, plant based diet. In the end, eating 100% plant based, without any animal product at all, was not for me. Even though I know how to do it, and not become deficient in some things such as b12, iron, calcium, and zinc. But mostly b12 is a common deficiency in vegans, and non vegans also.

100% plant based Vegan was not best suited for me. My testosterone was in the 600's after eating plant based vegan for a year. Which isn't low. And maybe even on the higher end of an almost 40 year old man.

But my testosterone is around 1000 now, since I added whole eggs back into my life. And I am now 41 and a half years old at the time of writing this now. And no, I do not take any steroids, or TRT, HRT prescriptions. My testosterone is high because my lifestyle. My diet. And my **MIND OVER MATTER.**

I consistently strive to become better tomorrow than I am today. I really try my best to live by this mantra. I want to share this part of me with you now, so that you can begin your own journey towards these same goals. Every single person on the planet would benefit from following this mantra. The world would be a better place if everyone did.

But few will. Very few will even entertain the thought of it. They would rather be distracted by all of the shiny objects that are flying in front of us at all times. Do not let that happen to you.

Create big goals for yourself. And stay consistent (in a healthy way), until you achieve, and exceed those goals. Our vitality should be number 1. The distractions in life are designed to make us put our vitality on the back burners. Some people never even put health on the bottom of their list to begin with. It is consistency that keeps us progressing. Life is short, and we should want to become better, and better each day, at living it.

I Have a Question to Ask You?

Why did you order this book?

Seriously, I really would like to know?

By the way, if you liked this book, if you can leave a review for me I would really appreciate that?

And in that review, I would love to know why you bought this book?

I have sold tens of thousands of my own personal self published books over the years, and even way more books that I have written under pen names. But for my own personal books, it always intrigues me why anyone would buy any of them?

It motivates me to continue writing them. And I really feel honored that I am able to have been a part of so many peoples lives.

Before I even started writing this book, I was trying to vision the avatar of the type of person who would order this book? And I couldn't narrow it down to just one. I think a wide variety of both men, and women are reading this book right now. My guess is that the majority of people reading this, would have a common goal of weight loss?

I don't think this is everyone. But I do think that the majority of both males and females reading this book, all ordered it because they themselves are wanting to lose weight, or get healthier in some sense. This is just my guess. Maybe some people ordered this book because of the personal story that I made very clear by the title. Some people love to read a real life happy ending story.

Whatever your reasons were for ordering this book are. I really hope that you come away more motivated, and driven to succeed in every aspect of your life. I know that by me writing it finally, and sharing a small piece of this big puzzle called my life. I am a stronger person afterwards. I feel good about the message that I portrayed throughout. And while I did not go into great detail about my personal life at this time. I really think that enough was told, for everyone reading it to understand where I was at in my life.

This book is actually supposed to be less about me, and more about what you can take, and apply to your life to make it the best life that you can possibly live. (The best, long life that you can possibly live.)

Personally, I have always been very good at not showing pain on the outside, while bleeding to death on the inside. This is just a trait that I have, and will more than likely never get rid of it completely. It is not just part of my personality. But I look the part of someone who has had it made in life.

Other than during those years when I let myself really go on the outside, I have always been able to keep all of my pain hidden from the world. Now, years later, when I look back at that time. I see myself, possibly subconsciously trying to match my outside, with what I had felt on the inside for so many years. I really think this could have been the case. I said earlier that our brains are so powerful. I could have been subconsciously trying to save my own life, by sharing with the world exactly what I thought of myself on the inside. I look at it as a positive, not a negative experience in my life.

I have been through so many negative experiences, that I am not sure if I can honestly turn them into a positive. But, this one I can. Because this one was my own doing. I got myself into, and out of this mess.

I was saying that I know that I look the part of someone who has been handed the good straw in life. I went through this as a kid. I never really looked the part of what I was. I always looked as if I was privileged, in comparison to some of the other kids in school, once I got into Jr High. But I was a poor kid. My mom was raising 4 kids by herself, on welfare for a long time, until she got trained for a job, that she is still at, and that she will retire from in a few years. If it wasn't for family, and friends helping out, we wouldn't have had a place to live probably. In fact, at one time, we had 3 other poor families living in our 3 bedroom house. 19 people in one little 3 bedroom home.

In elementary school, I was looked at as kind of one of the poor kids. I got the free lunches, and all that. My shoes were from Payless, and clothes from K Mart, the other cheap outlets. Crazy how even little kids judge other kids by their brand of clothes and shoes. It is actually very sad that we as a 1st world society are that petty, that young.

Anyways...

My elementary school experience, was completely different than my Jr High experience. The elementary school I went to was in a decent area. More kids parents had jobs at least. There were even a few upper middle class kids. But mostly middle classers who work. I was one of the few poor kids who went to this school. It was easy to tell the difference between poor and middle class at this time.

The Jr High I got sent to was not quite filled with middle class family kids. It was filled with kids who are also on welfare, like myself. But this school was in the heart of a predominantly black ghetto, where my dad was raised. My grandparents still live there in the same house. They will die there. It used to be Crip territory. It still might be now, although things have changed for the better over there. The gangs aren't what they were 30 years ago.

The school I went to was mostly black kids. And most of them were gang members from birth. They were born into it. They knew nothing else. There were a few Mexican gangs too. But mostly a wide variety of Crips, and some Blood street gangs. All in one little Jr High School. There were some hardcore kids at this school when I went there. They all had a prison mentality at a very young age. The schools vibe was like being locked up in prison.

People who look like me don't exactly get accepted very easily by poor people. And I am technically Mexican. But I don't fit the mold of a thug Mexican that would be accepted by their crowd. I didn't want to either. I never tried to act like a thug. I always stayed far away from that life, even though I seen family members run towards it. Unfortunately they fit the mold. So they are accepted by others who also fit the mold. I am very lucky that I didn't fit the mold, and look the part. Or I may not be writing this book today. I would have probably had to join in with them, and prove myself to them too. But luckily, they didn't want me, and I didn't want them.

So I go from being one of the poor kids in elementary school. To being looked at as a privileged white boy (even though I am Mexican), who has had everything handed to me in life. It was weird, because I was just as poor as everyone else at that school. I had the free lunch cards just like they all did. I was raised for a good chunk of my life on welfare.

Ever since then I realized that I was always being judged by what I looked like. I am so glad that I never really tried to be anything other than myself. I didn't try and harden myself up, and put on an act, in order to impress certain thugs around me. I would have felt so stupid for that if I had. And would if it worked? I would not be here writing this book today. I could even be dead.

Many kids that I went to Jr High with aren't even alive now. Several kids that I went to school with were killed before they even got out of their teen years. I remember there was a thing going on with certain Mexican gangs that were fighting with other Mexicans. They were slitting each others throats. I knew a lot of kids from school who got their throats slit before they even turned 20 years old. Some lived through it, and some did not.

If I ever can get myself to write that book on my own suicidal fantasies since a very young age. I would possibly tell some crazy stories from this time in my childhood that would shock some people. As of right now, I am not feeling like writing it. I won't write anything that can affect my future progress in life. I am about moving onward and upward. I don't want to go backwards, and get stuck in time warp. We shall see if I ever get around to doing it. As of now, I am not interested in telling this part of my life, through anything other than my music lyrics. But we shall see, as time goes on. I wrote this book didn't I?

Blood Work – How Often Do You Have it Done?

Test	Result	Flag	Units	Reference Range	
Neutrophils Absolute	2.68		10*3/uL	1.50 - 7.00	
Lymphs Absolute	1.57		10*3/uL	0.90 - 3.50	
Monos Absolute	0.38		10*3/uL	0.10 - 1.10	
Eosinophils Absolute	0.08		10*3/uL	0.00 - 0.80	
Basophils Absolute	0.03		10*3/uL	0.00 - 0.30	
Vitamin D 25-OH, Total	128.0	H	ng/mL	30.0 - 100.0	WPML

```
       Vitamin D status      25-OH Vitamin D
       Deficiency            < 10 ng/mL
       Insufficiency         10-29 ng/mL
       Sufficiency           30-100 ng/mL
       Toxicity              >100 ng/mL
```

Lipid Panel					WPML
Cholesterol, Total	126		mg/dL	0 - 199	
Cholesterol-HDL	51		mg/dL	>39	
Cholesterol/HDL Cholesterol Ratio (Calc)	2.47		Ratio	<5.60	
Non-HDL Cholesterol (Calc.)	75		mg/dL	<130	
Triglycerides	70		mg/dL	<150	
LDL (Calc.)	61		mg/dL	<100	

LDL calculations are valid only when Triglycerides is less than 400 mg/dL.

VLDL (Calc.)	14		mg/dL	<40	
TESTOSTERONE, F/T WITH SHBG					
TESTOSTERONE	947	H	ng/dL	300 - 890	WPML
SEX HORM BIND GLOBULIN	83	H	nmol/L	18 - 66	WPML
Testosterone, Free, (Calc.)	114.3		pg/mL	35.0 - 180.0	WPML
Testosterone, Free, %	1.21		%	1.00 - 2.70	WPML

**NOTE: The result is based on the formula derived from the estimation of Free Testosterone in serum (J. Clin Endocrinol Metab 84:3666-3672,1999)

I really wish that I was getting blood work done during this weight loss. Before, during, and after. I barely started getting my blood drawn a few years ago. I will get my blood drawn each year for sure from now on. And even sometimes more than once a year for some things. For me, my testosterone, vitamin d, b12, and lipids, are what I want to see perfect levels of. Not that I don't want perfect levels of everything else. Its just, if these are great, then everything else seems to be great as well. If you have not checked out my little YouTube channel for these books, do so. I show my full panel blood test. My channel is Dexter the vEGGan.

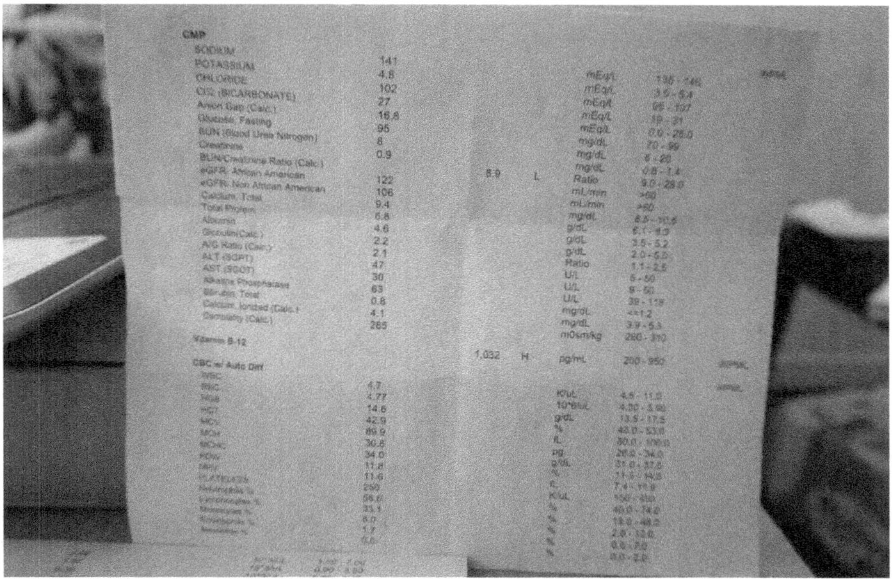

I am 41 years old. And I am honestly healthier now, than I was at 18 - 21, when I was amateur kickboxing, and in very good shape. But I was relying on good genetics, youth, and more good genetics, and youth. This might sound mean. But don't even listen to anyone on the internet in their 20's, who try and act like they know about health. And even most people on the internet in their 30's. Heck, even most people on the internet no matter what their age is. If they are marketing themselves as an expert, or guru in the field. Be cautious, and understand that you are not always being told everything about them and their own health. Because many of them aren't actually healthy.

So many males, and females online are taking "stuff", in order to give them that little bit better than the average person's body. None of them would dare to show their full panel blood work on video. It would be a complete mess. And also show what kin d of "stuff" they are taking.

I would tell people, not to even take advice from someone about health who does not show their blood tests regularly. And not just show small parts of it. Show the entire blood test. Be proud of it. I have not seen anyone who does this so far? Maybe they are out there. But they are not at the higher levels of heath *guruism.*

I can write an entire book about this subject. And maybe one day I will. But the point of bringing up my blood work here, is so that you can see the importance of regular blood testing. Like once a year is great. You don't need to be a freak and test specific things throughout the year. Once a year is good to know where you are at in your general health. I wish that I was testing yearly a long time ago. Especially during this time when I lost all of this weight.

And also understand that one blood test isn't always going to give you definitive answers to all of your problems, and ailments. But they are good to use as a base to work from. Find a good Doctor that lets you see, and keep your test results. Some won't even let you see them.

For me this past year, my personal goal was to keep my vitamin d up around 100 ng/ml. I knew that if my vitamin d is up high, so will be my testosterone. Getting it there, and keeping it there are two different things. My focus is on keeping these levels high throughout the remainder of my life.

I have no clue what my testosterone, and vitamin d levels were during this weight loss period, because I did not test them. I didn't even think about any of that stuff then. But I imagine that they were both nowhere near what they are today, more than a decade later.

I set the bar very high for myself. I plan on keeping myself at least 20 years younger than I am. It is a lifestyle choice that I encourage everyone to consider making. Most people don't know how to even care a little bit about their own health. And if they eventually are forced to because of illness. They really don't want to. They would rather be doing something more entertaining to them.

I do my best to be an example of the opposite of that. That is all that I can do. I only can focus on my longevity. And live what I say that I live. I am not anyone's leader, or guru. I don't want to be either. I just want to focus on my own self. And if that motivates others to do the same, that is what makes me feel good.

Check these other books out.

Before you shut this book, I want you to check out some of these other books by myself. Some of them may even be FREE in eBook. You can find them all for sure on Amazon. And some of them are also sold on other platforms as well.

I have 3 author pages on Amazon that you can check out under – Dexter Mason, Dexter Poin, & Dexter Lives. I actually have more than 3, but those are three that you can check out, and find more of my books, and short eBooks.

Don't forget to drop me a review for this book. I really appreciate that more than you know. I don't purchase fake reviews like everyone else in this business does. (oops did I let a cat out of a bag? It is too true though.) So I really appreciate all reviews, as I know how hard the real ones are to get out of real people who have busy lives.

Also, do not forget to come hang out with me on some social media platforms.
Instagram - @dextersworld
YouTube – Dexter the vEGGan & Dexter Lives(my music channel)
Facebook – Dexter Lives

The Healthiest
MEAL PREP
Guide on
EARTH
Eat Exactly Like Me For Just 10 Days!
Dexter Mason
Reduce Inflammation
Reverse Aging
Rethink the Entire Concept of Food
Recipes & Meal Planning Videos Inside!
For Males & Females

HEALTHY EATING
on
a
BUDGET

Dexter Poin

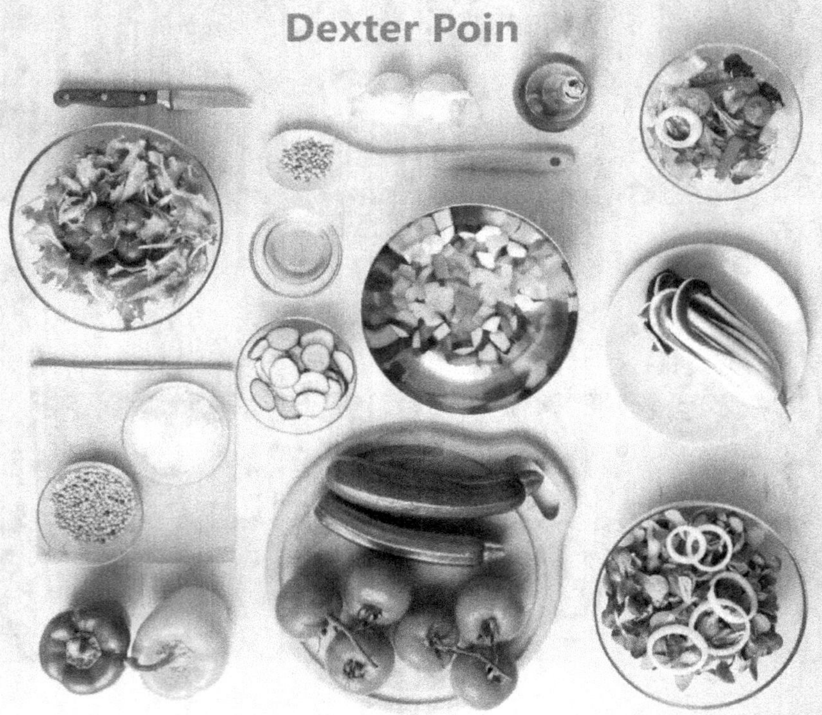

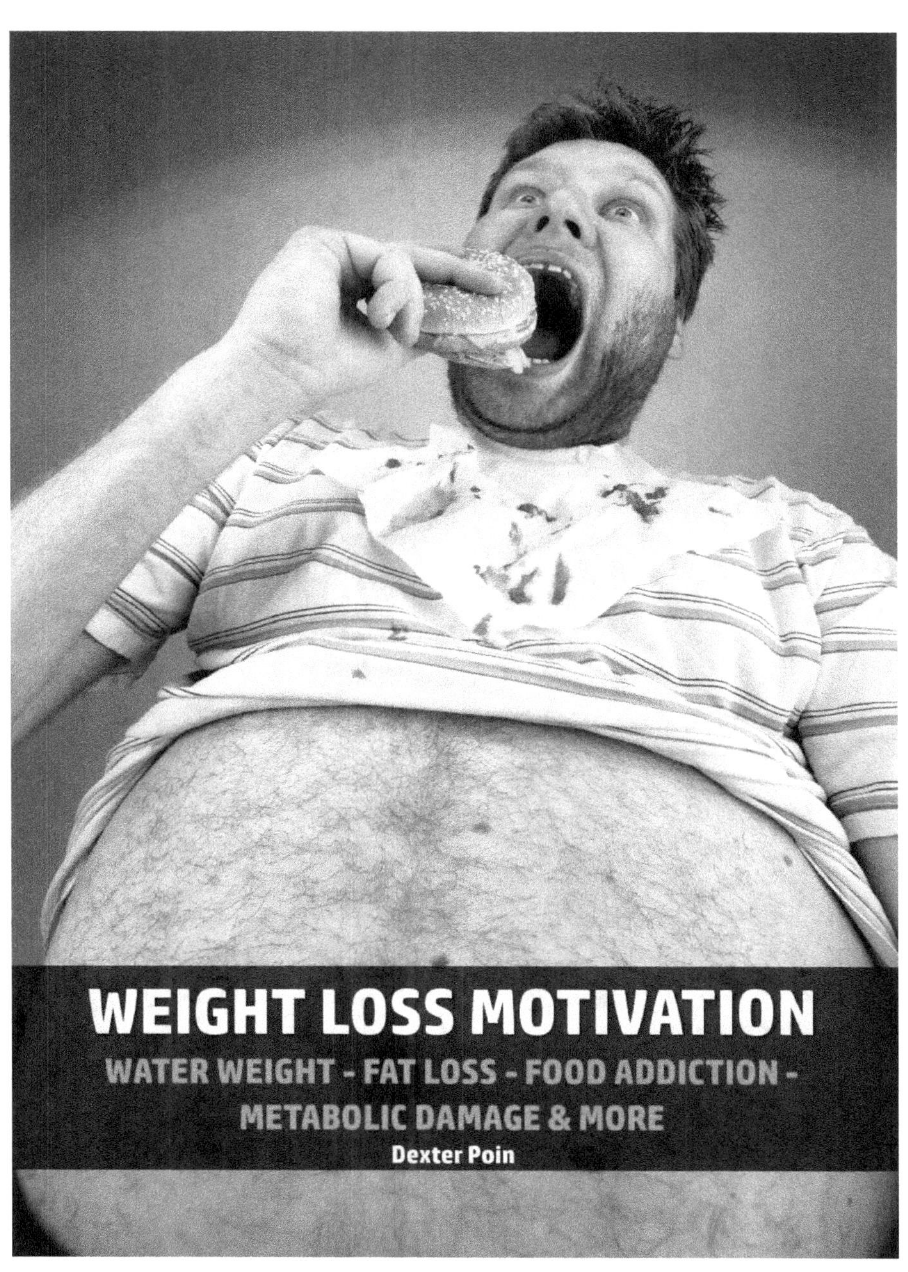

WEIGHT LOSS MOTIVATION
WATER WEIGHT - FAT LOSS - FOOD ADDICTION -
METABOLIC DAMAGE & MORE
Dexter Poin

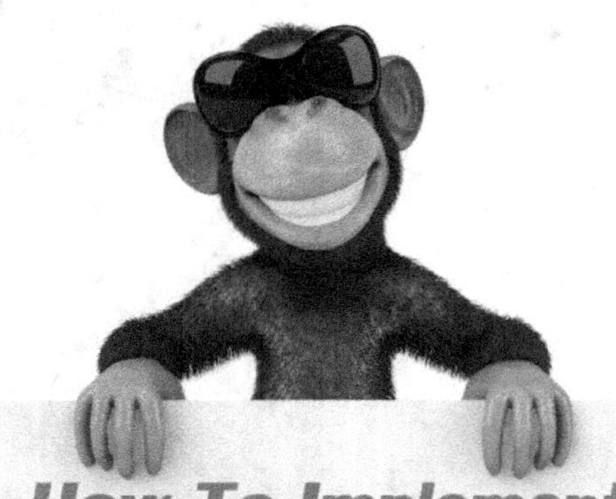
How To Implement
Raw Foods Into Your
Life in the Real World

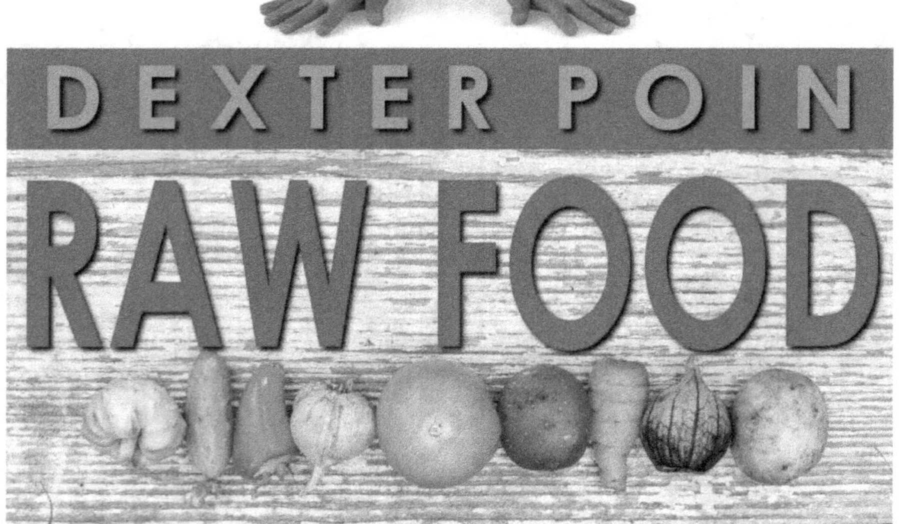
DEXTER POIN
RAW FOOD

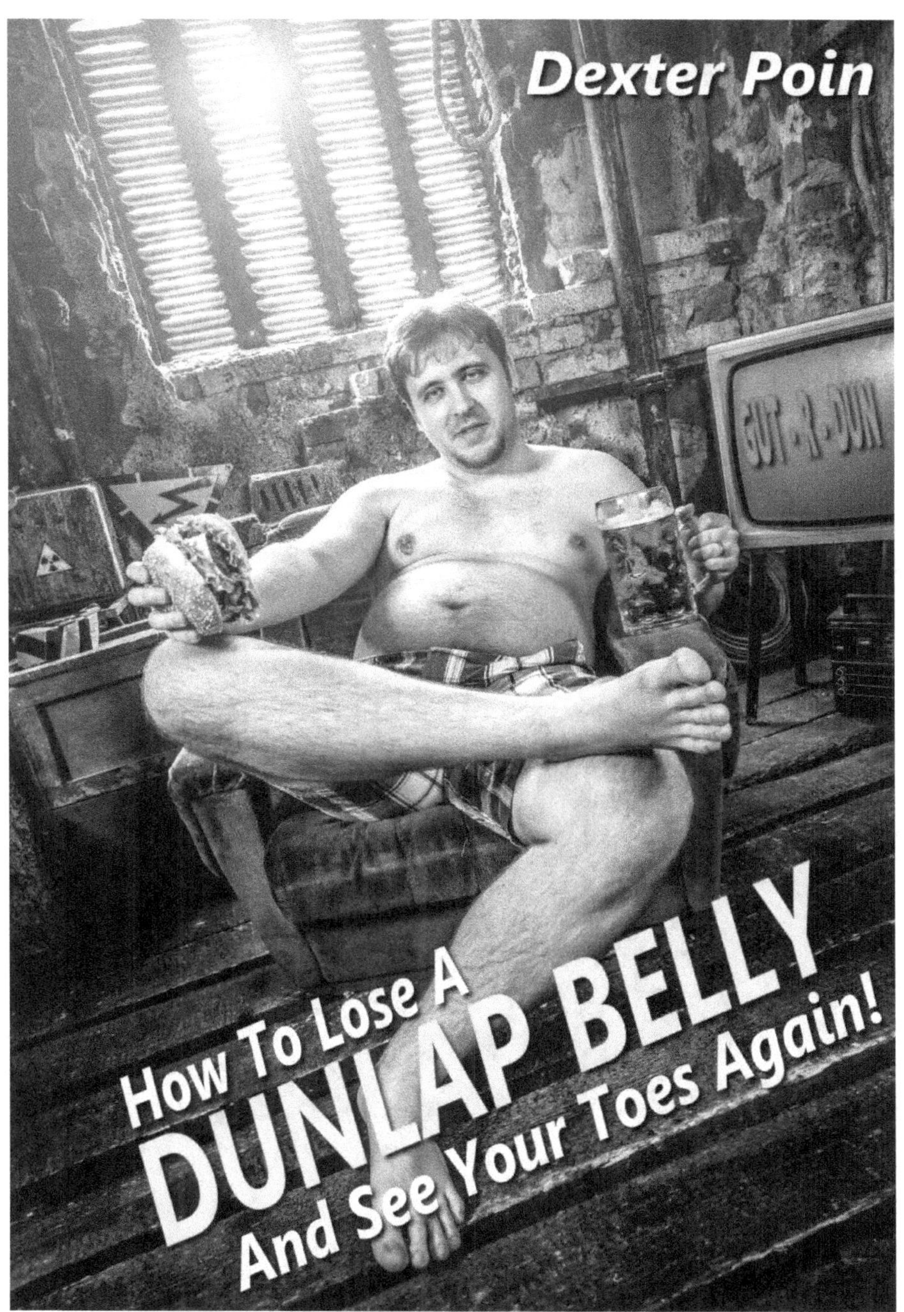
Dexter Poin
How To Lose A
DUNLAP BELLY
And See Your Toes Again!
GUT-R-DUN

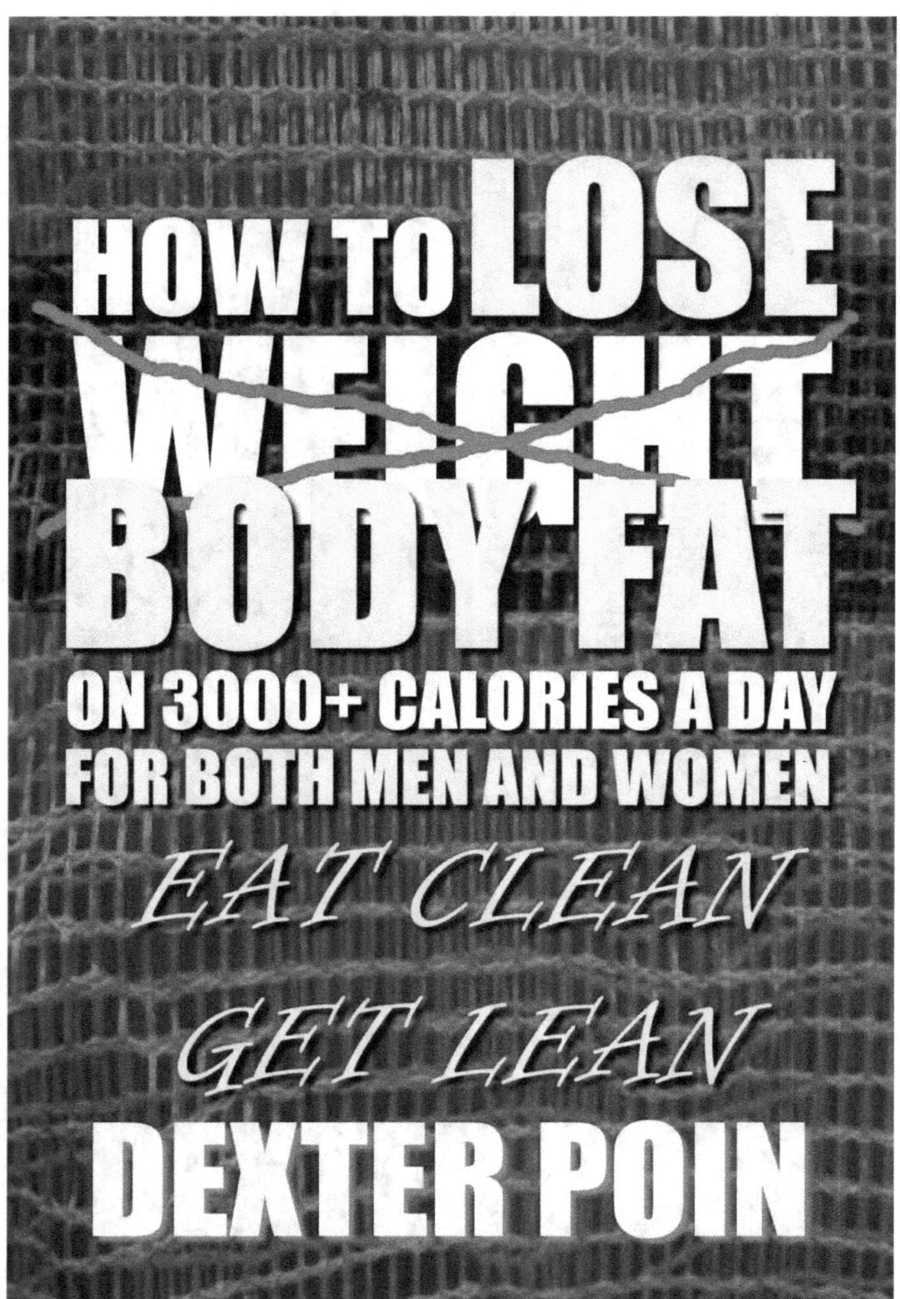

HOW TO LOSE
WEIGHT
BODY FAT
ON 3000+ CALORIES A DAY
FOR BOTH MEN AND WOMEN
EAT CLEAN
GET LEAN
DEXTER POIN

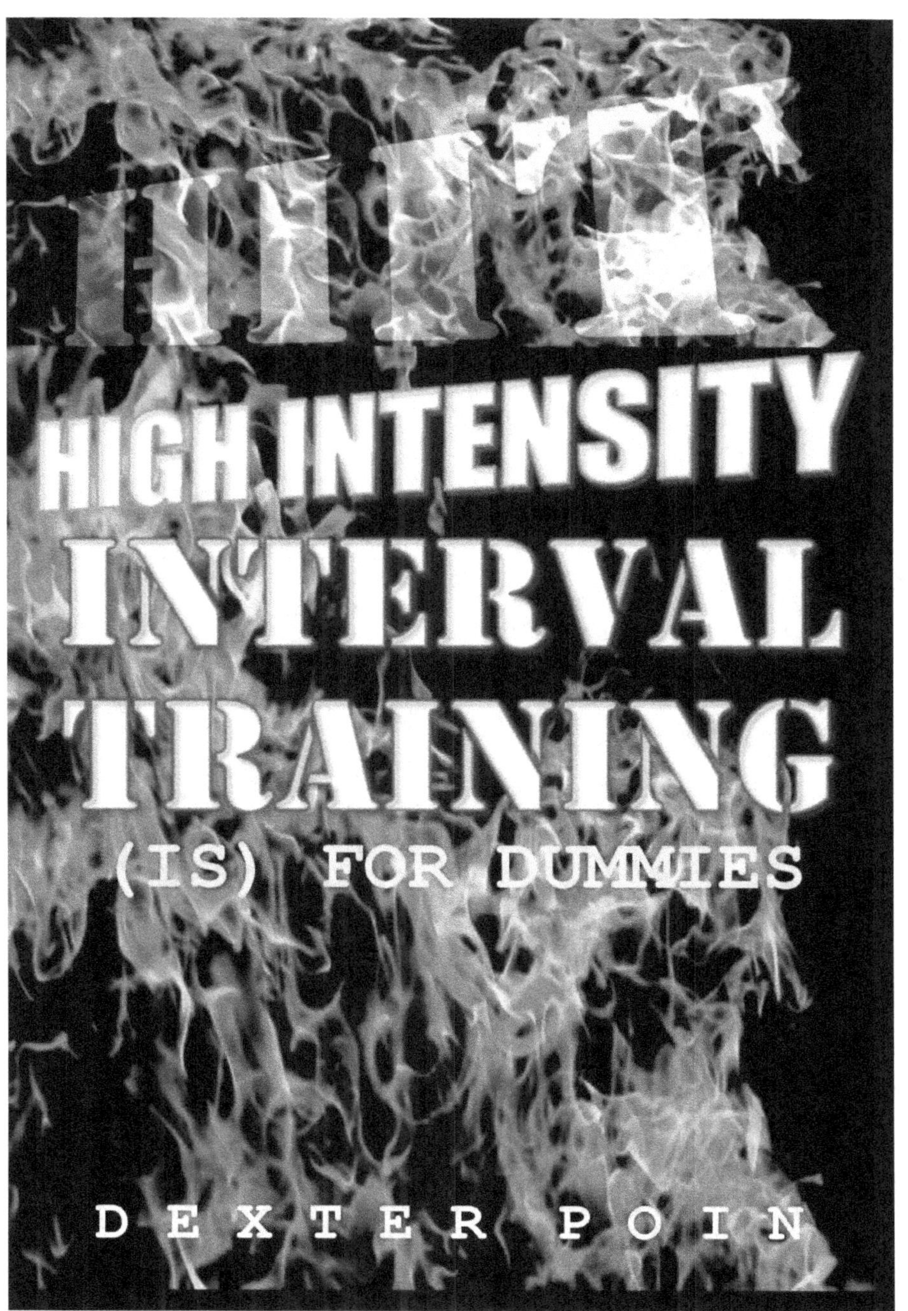

HIIT
HIGH INTENSITY
INTERVAL
TRAINING
(IS) FOR DUMMIES
DEXTER POIN

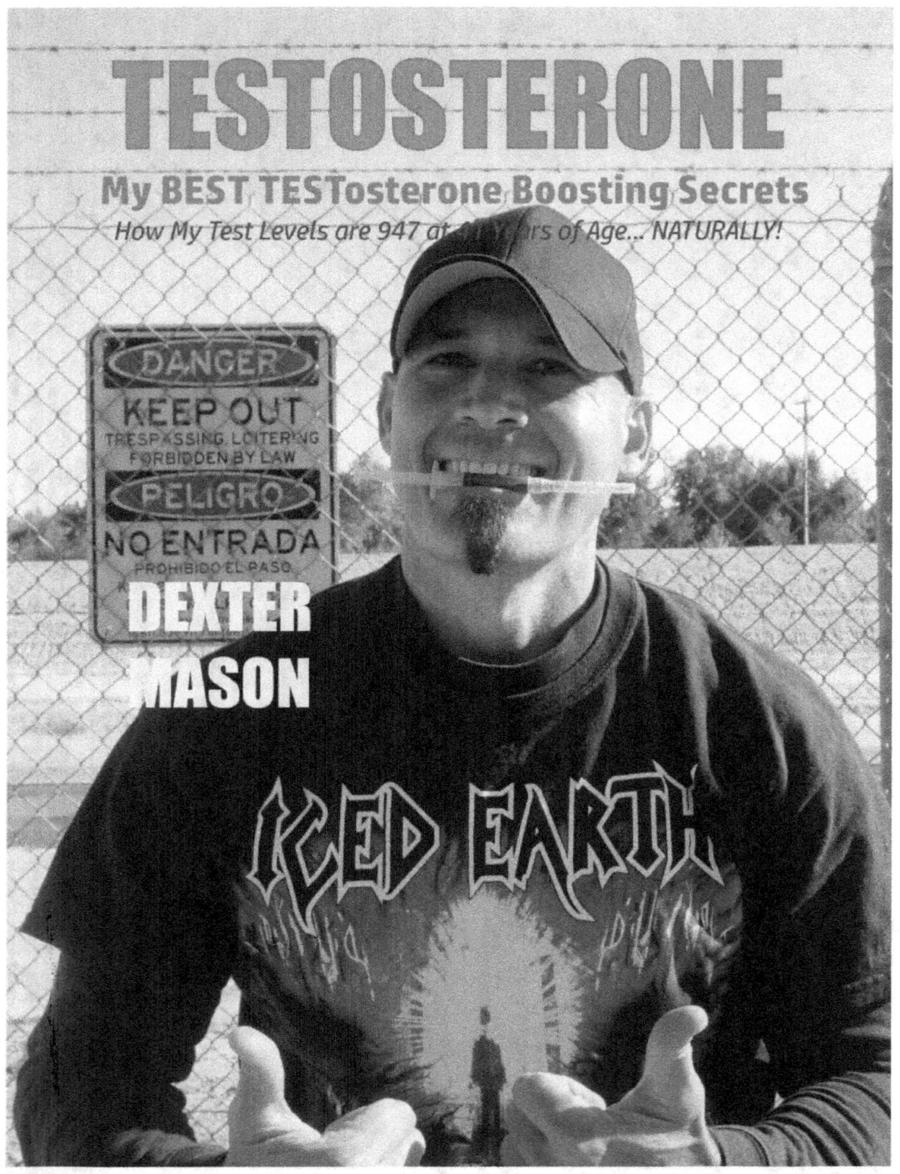

Men, as of right now, I have not yet written this life changing book yet. And I may never even write it. If you want me to put this invaluable information together, you have got to let me know? Get on my email list too.

Links are inside of my eBooks. In the description of my YouTube channel videos. Or you can email me at dextermason77@gmail.com and I can email you a clickable link, if you cannot find one in those places.

There is nothing out there as real world as this on the market. Nothing even close. I am 41 years old, with a testosterone level around 1000 at all times. And I do not take any synthetic testosterone, or even any test boosting supplements. And I show all of my blood work to prove it.

If this interests you, find out more by going and finding all of the videos, and links where I am talking about it. I need enough people to want this, or I won't provide it. I just do not have the time to. I will continue living it though.

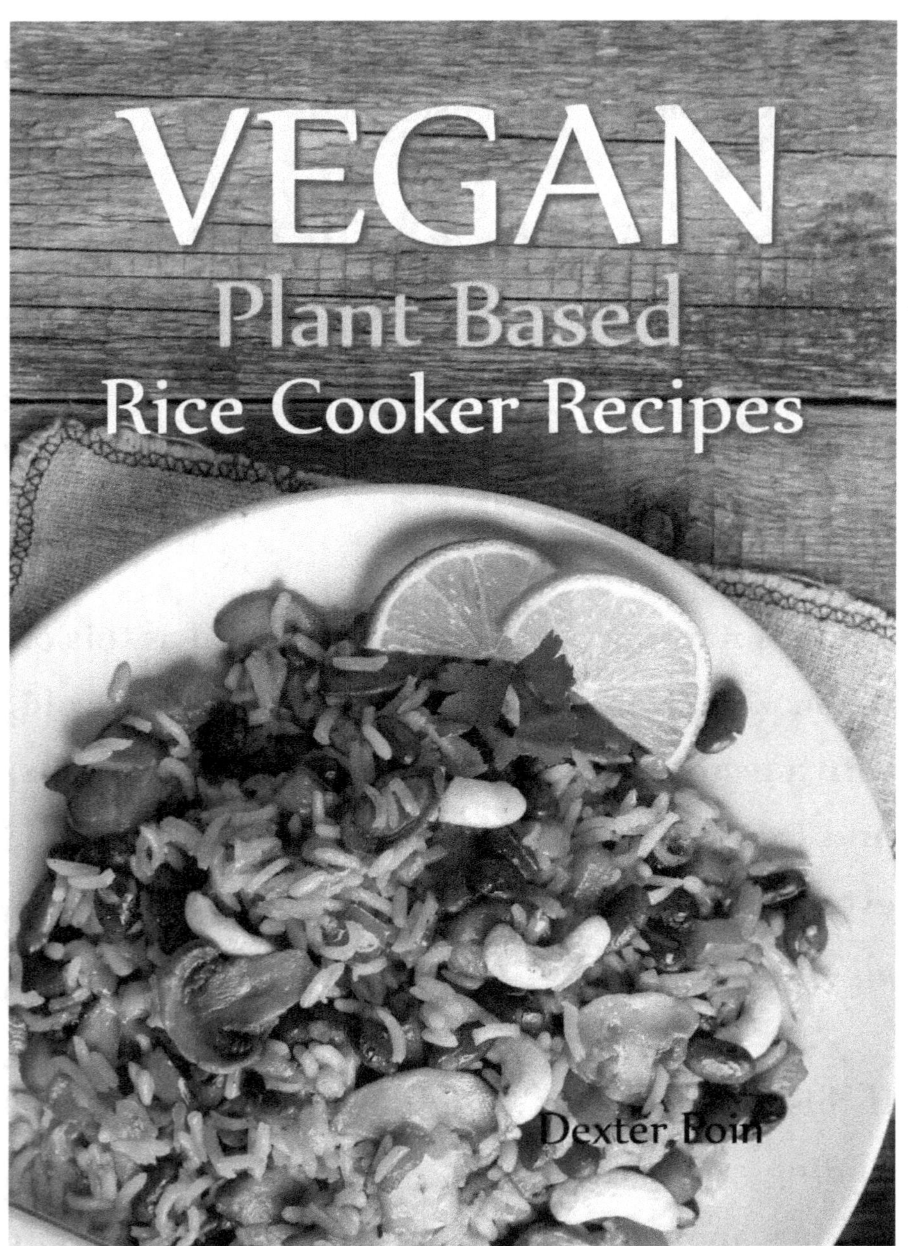

VEGAN
Plant Based
Rice Cooker Recipes
Dexter Boin

DEXTER POIN
RICE
50+ RICE COOKER RECIPES
RICE
100% VEGAN APPROVED!
BABY
QUICK AND EASY
COOKING FOR A HEALTHY
WAY OF LIFE!

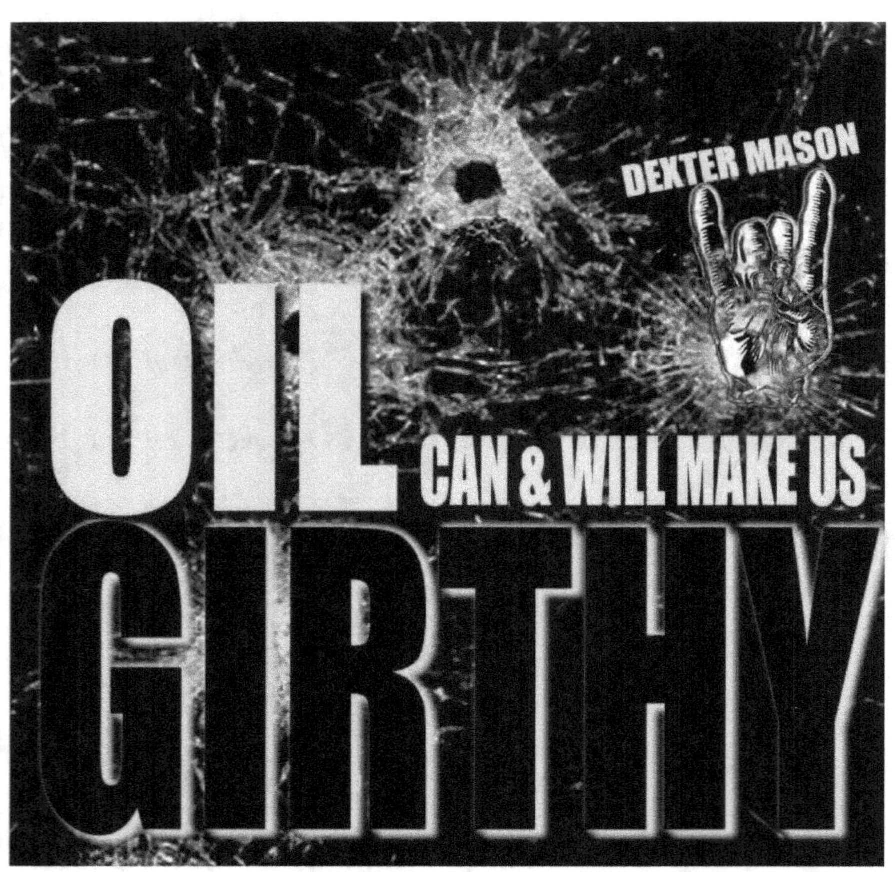

DEXTER MASON
OIL
CAN & WILL MAKE US
GIRTHY

HOW
DEXTER MASON
ADDICTION
TURNS INTO
OBSESSION

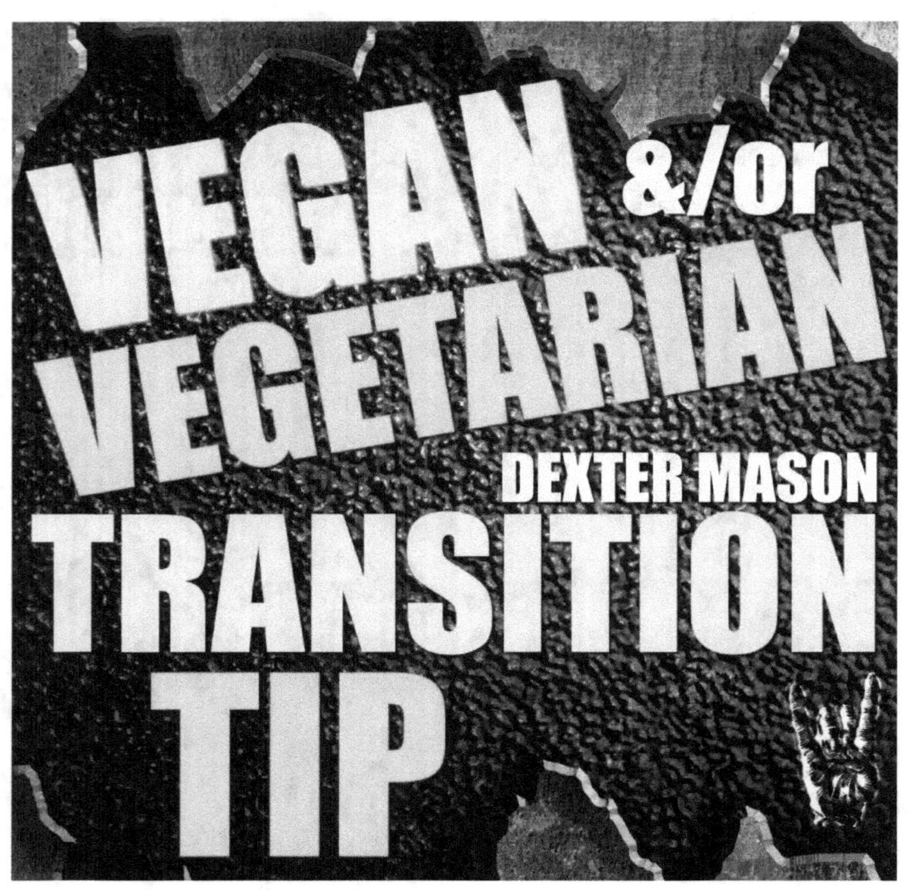

VEGAN &/or
VEGETARIAN
DEXTER MASON
TRANSITION
TIP

DEXTER LIVES

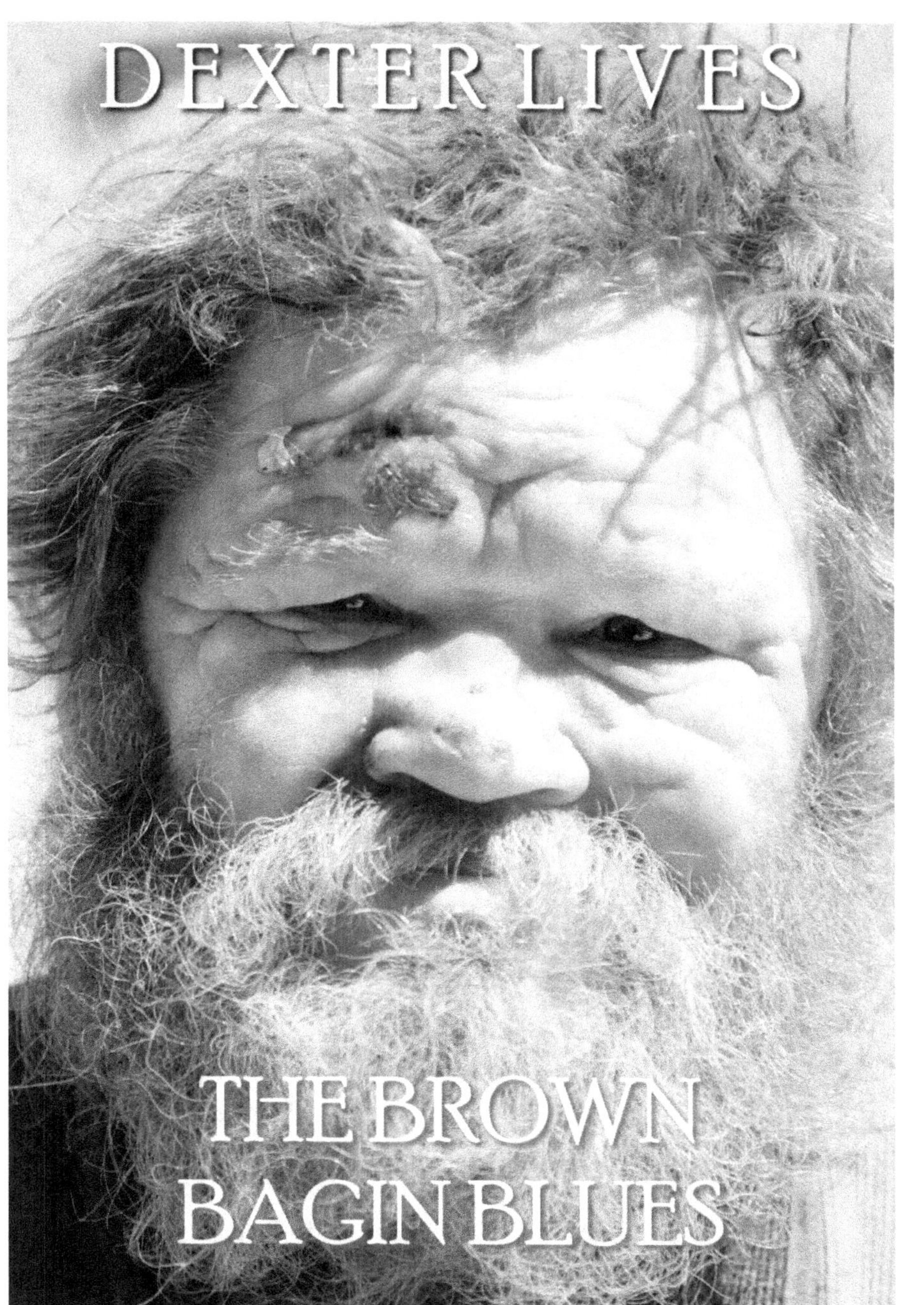

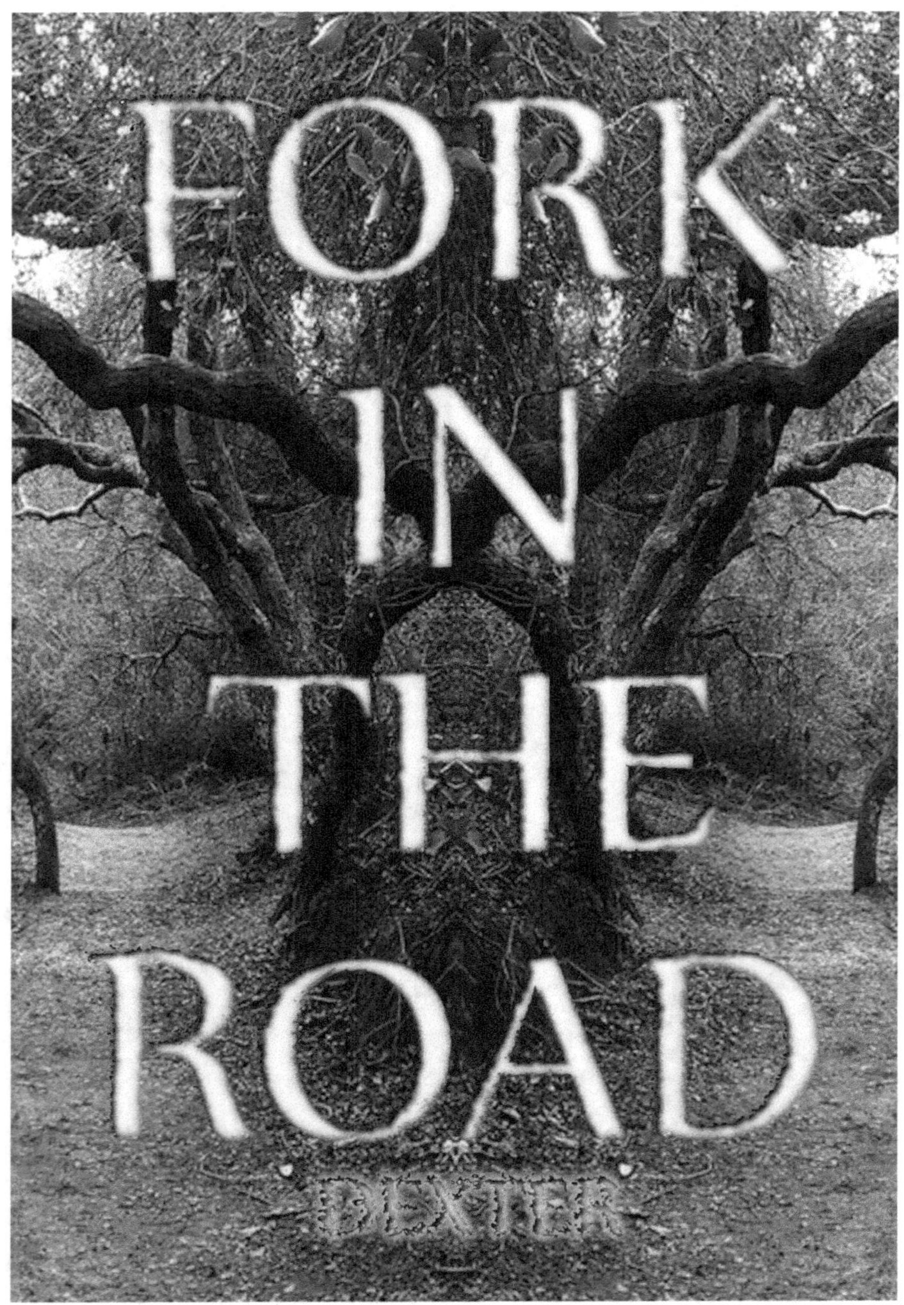

FORK
IN
THE
ROAD
DEXTER

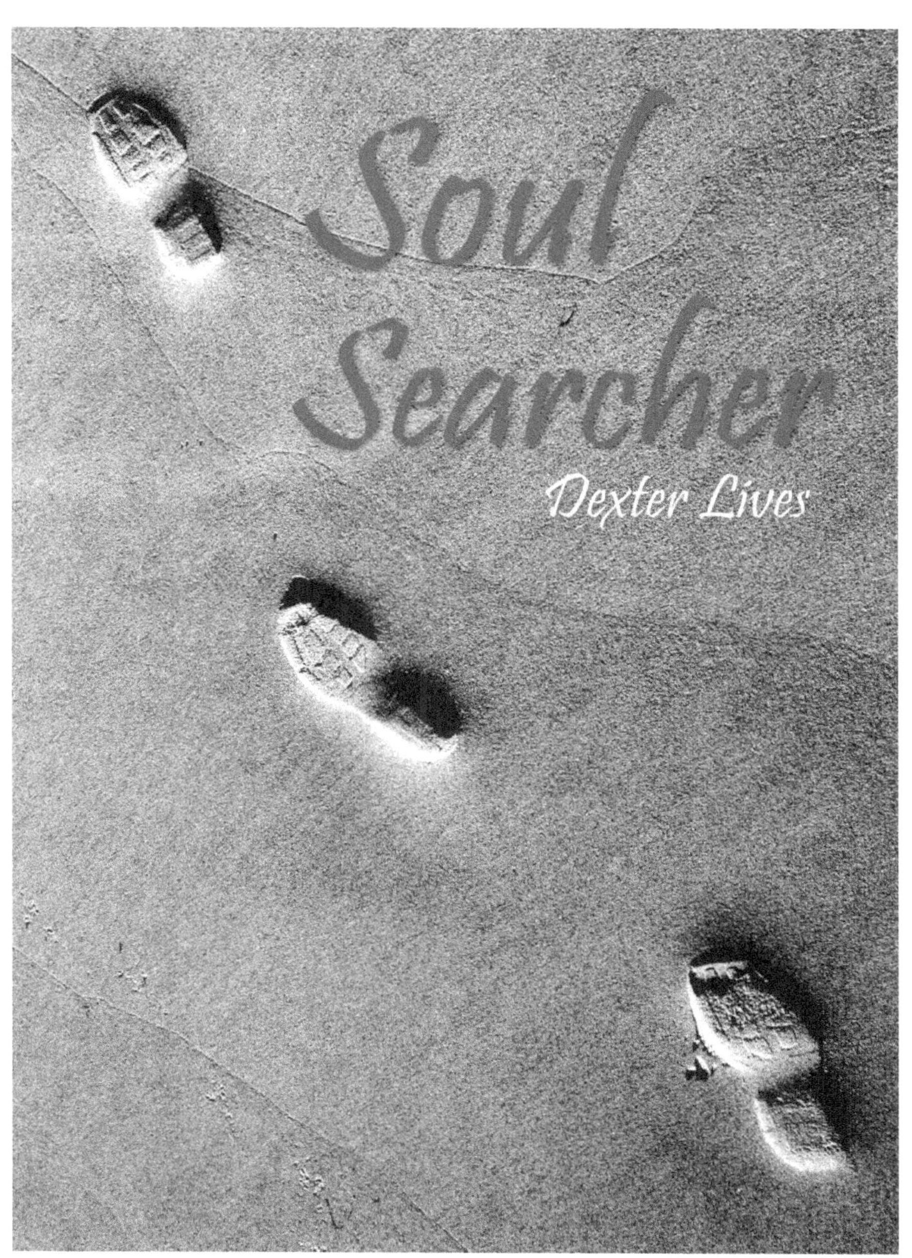
Soul
Searcher
Dexter Lives

Look below

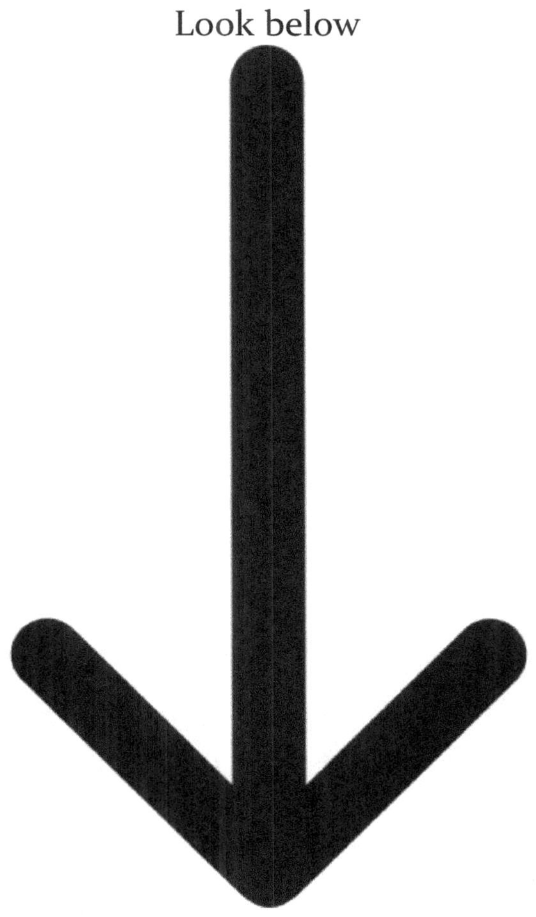

I want you to THRIVE until you reach that number in age!